Community health workers in national programmes

Just another pair of hands?

Community health workers in national programmes:
Just another pair of hands?

Gill Walt (editor) with
Lucy Gilson, Kris Heggenhougen, Thutego Knudsen, Lucas Owuor-Omondi, Myrtle Perera, David Ross, Ligia Salazar and Sarah Malins

OPEN UNIVERSITY PRESS
MILTON KEYNES · PHILADELPHIA

Open University Press
Celtic Court
22 Ballmoor
Buckingham MK18 1XW

and
1900 Frost Road, Suite 101
Bristol, PA 19007, USA

First Published 1990

British Library Cataloguing in Publication Data

Community health workers in national programmes: just another pair of hands?
1. Developing Countries. Health service
I. Walt, Gill.   II. Gilson, Lucy
362.1'09172'4

ISBN 0 335 15433 6
ISBN 0 335 15432 8 (pbk)

Library of Congress Cataloging-in-Publication Data

Community health workers in national development programmes: just another
pair of hands?/Gill Walt, editor, with Lucy Gilson ... [et al.].
  p. cm.
ISBN 0-335-15433-6   ISBN 0-335-15432-8 (pbk.)
1. Community health services 2. Community health aides.
I. Walt, Gillian.
RA427.C618   1990
362-1'2--dc20   89-71096
                                                                          CIP

Typeset by Burns & Smith, Derby
Printed in Great Britain by Biddles Limited, Guildford & Kings Lynn

Contents

List of tables
and figures

Figures

Preface

The journey from the nearest town took five hours, half of it on a sandy road past nothing but salt pans, baobab trees and the odd fleeting glimpse of a springbok. We arrived at the health clinic in Maun – a large village of about 70,000 people – just before noon. The morning's work was almost over. A nurse was taking a woman's blood pressure, a few mothers and babies were waiting patiently to see another nurse. Outside a small group was sitting under a tree, receiving nutrition education.

The chief nurse was welcoming, and when we explained why we had come her enthusiasm was uninhibited. 'Family welfare educators?' she exclaimed, indicating the woman who was sweeping the clinic floor. 'We couldn't do without them! It's wonderful to have extra pairs of hands in a busy clinic like this!'

Family welfare educators (FWEs) are Botswana's community health workers (CHWs). They receive sixteen weeks' training and are supposed to spend half their time in the community and the other half assisting in the health clinics. But everywhere we went in Botswana we were told – even by the FWEs themselves – that in practice they spend most of their time in the health facilities rather than visiting homes in their communities. It seemed that the FWEs' role had changed from what had originally been intended, and that they had become 'just another pair of hands' at the primary level of the health service.

This book is the result of research which set out to explore what had happened to CHWs in national programmes. We knew that there were many positive examples of small, often non-governmental organizations, training local people as CHWs, frequently with stunning results such as lowering the infant mortality rate, and improving nutrition. We knew that these examples (and the impetus of the primary health care (PHC) approach) had stimulated many countries to set up CHW programmes on a national scale. We knew, too, that these programmes had expanded throughout the 1970s on a wave of enthusiasm and optimism which saw

CHWs in many roles: as liberators, pillars of health for all, the corner-stone of primary health care, extenders of services. But we also knew that, by the mid-1980s, many questions were being raised about the value and costs of national programmes.

Critics of CHW programmes pointed out that they were often inhibitors of community care rather than liberators; that reviews of CHWs had revealed great weaknesses in many programmes, especially in their supervision and support; that training had been suspended in Jamaica and Colombia, and numbers trained had been cut in Botswana largely for financial reasons; that over fifty years of training CHWs in Peru had left little trace; and that even China's 'barefoot doctor' programme, once the inspiration to all, had been modified by the early 1980s.

Where did this leave CHW programmes? What remained true was that in many countries there were rural and peri-urban populations with very poor access to preventive or curative health services. There were insufficient financial resources to train doctors or nurses to serve in these areas, and anyway medical personnel were often reluctant to be posted to peripheral health facilities.

In 1986 a multi-disciplinary team from the Evaluation and Planning Centre for Health Care (EPC), London School of Hygiene and Tropical Medicine, approached the UK Overseas Development Administration for support for a research study on policy and practice in national CHW programmes. Such a study could inform policy-makers – both national and international – on the options for future commitment to these programmes. The major objective of the study was to re-examine the implementation of national CHW programmes, looking at the policy, planning and management implications of this experience. The EPC team consisted of a sociologist, an anthropologist, an epidemiologist and, in the final year, an economist. An important ethos directing the research was that it should be done collaboratively, with national partners taking an active role in the research design, operation and analysis.

This book disseminates the findings from that study. It starts by looking at the context of changing health policies over the past four decades, the emphasis given to PHC in the 1970s and the resulting confusion about who is the community health worker. The second part of the book addresses the crucial issues about national CHW programmes: what tasks and skills CHWs have; their place in the health system; and the costs and financing of CHW programmes. A chapter on the problems of evaluating CHW programmes is followed by detailed case studies from Botswana, Colombia and Sri Lanka. Finally, if CHW programmes are in difficulties it is not because they cannot deliver, but because the support that makes them effective is all too often absent. The last chapter attempts to look beyond the problems currently being faced, to see how CHW programmes can be made to work more successfully.

A book like this is the result of many people's enthusiasm and inputs.

Parts I, II and IV are written largely by Gill Walt (Chapters 1–4, 10), and Lucy Gilson (Chapter 5). Part III, apart from the introductory Chapter 6 by Gill Walt, was the combined effort of many. The Botswana case study involved Lucas Owuor-Omondi and Thutego Knudsen of the Health Research Unit, Ministry of Health, Gaborone, as well as David Ross, Lucy Gilson and Gill Walt from the EPC. The Colombian case study involved Ligia Salazar, Esmeralda Burbano and Virginia Trujillo of CIMDER, Universidad del Valle, Cali, with Kris Heggenhougen and David Ross from the EPC. Finally, the Sri Lankan study was the work of Myrtle Perera, of the Marga Institute, Colombo, with Gill Walt and Kris Heggenhougen of the EPC. At early stages colleagues in the EPC commented on various aspects of the research. The book gained greatly from Sarah Malins' editing skills and picture research.

However, although particular people are responsible for different chapters, the ideas and, in particular, the conclusions, are everyone's: most people involved in the study read and commented on all chapters, and some suggested detailed and useful alterations to the text. The sum, we hope, is greater than the parts.

Acknowledgements

The study on which this book is based was jointly supported by the UK Overseas Development Administration; the Director General's special fund for health systems research in Botswana; the Maternal Child Health Division of the Colombian Ministry of Health, and the Centre for Multi-disciplinary Development Research (CIMDER) of the Universidad del Valle, Cali; and the Marga Institute and Health Education Bureau, Colombo, Sri Lanka.

Many participated in the development and implementation of the project, including community health workers and community members who invited us into their homes and gave freely of their time. Their collaboration was greatly appreciated. To them and others named below, our special thanks.

In Botswana:
T. Maganu, N. Ngcongco, W. Manyeneng, P. Khulumani, R. Mandevu, R. Diseko, W. Osei, D. Mosiieman, B. Pilane, J. Pederson, J. van Dam, S. Anderson, C. Isayi, *Ministry of Health*
P. Siele, L. Molamu, *Ministry of Local Government and Lands*
P. Sieben, P. Rojas, *World Health Organization*
G. Pfau, consultant
S. Kimaryo, *UNICEF*
The health team at Mochudi clinic, the Maun district health team, and all the district health teams who assisted with the distribution of the national family welfare educators' questionnaire.

In Colombia:
E. Burbano and V. Trujillo who did most of the field research, J. Saravia, R. Otero and other colleagues in CIMDER, Cali
M. Palacio Hurtado, O. Rojas, H. Perdamo, W. Rodríguez, L. A. Valero, C. Gross, E. Sánchez, G. Calixto, *Ministry of Health, Bogotá*

I. Durana, A. Ordónez Plaja, D. Bersh, H. A. Gómez, R. Guerrero, H. Valencia, J. Rodríquez, K. Mokate, I. Lara, A. Meija

In Sri Lanka:
G. Gunatilleke, *Marga Institute*
M. Perera, L. Abergunawardene, *Health Education Bureau*
M. de Silva, *Family Health Bureau*
A. Meegama, H. Wijemanne, *UNICEF*
J. Fernando, R. Jayasuriya, *Ministry of Health*
The MOH and public health team at Galle, Mawanella and Anuradhapura

In London:
Colleagues in the Evaluation and Planning Centre, London School of Hygiene and Tropical Medicine

PART I
Background

1 | Community health workers: the evolution of a concept

Before 1975 neither the words 'community health workers' (CHWs) nor 'primary health care' (PHC) were generally used, even among health professionals. Today they are common parlance, although conceptual and definitional differences abound: some people even describe CHW programmes as synonymous with PHC. Indeed, over the last decade CHW programmes have expanded enormously. How did this change occur? Why did thinking about health policy shift in favour of CHWs and PHC? Different types of CHW had existed for years on a small scale. Why the flurry of activity in the 1970s and 1980s?

To understand how the concept of the CHW was promoted internationally and adopted nationally, we need to look at the context within which changing ideas about health, and especially primary health care, took place. In this chapter, therefore, we set the context by distinguishing five areas of influence and changing ideas about health, although any such division is to some extent arbitrary. Policy change occurs as the result of a complex sequence of events and ideas not necessarily distinguishable over time. However, for analytical purposes, it is possible to focus on five areas:

1 Changing ideas about poverty, health and development
2 Concern about population growth
3 Disillusion with the medical care model
4 Community involvement and self-care
5 Activities and policies of the international organizations

We will consider each of these separately before going on in the next chapter to look at the concept of CHWs and at governments' attempts to introduce CHW programmes.

Changing ideas about poverty, health and development

The current emphasis on health as an aspect of development can be seen partly as a reaction against the neglect of health (and other social dimensions of welfare) in the literature on development which was produced in the 1950s and 1960s. This emanated mainly from the developed countries, as a guide to economic and social policy in the newly independent countries of the Third World. Any simple generalization about this literature must be to some extent misleading, neglecting the differences between writers and perhaps exaggerating the effect their theories had on the actual policies of developing countries. But from the point of view of their successors in the 1970s, the earlier writers appear to have some common characteristics which led them to neglect the social aspects of development.

The early post-Second World War development theories stressed the overriding importance of investment in the physical elements of national growth – industry, roads, dams and so on – and saw health and other social services such as education as non-productive consumption sectors. Thus government money expended on such services was a dissipation of national savings.

In order to counter such arguments, and rationalize expenditure on health, some studies attempted to demonstrate that changes in the health of populations would result in increased productivity and therefore rising per capita incomes. Empirical findings were, however, contradictory (Grosse and Harkavy 1980). For example, studies in St Lucia showed no effect on production when workers suffering from schistosomiasis were treated (Weisbrod *et al.* 1974), although a similar study in Indonesia concluded that workers without hookworm performed better than those with the parasite (Basta and Churchill 1974). There were also numerous methodological problems with the studies (Beenstock 1980).

Other studies pointed to accumulating evidence of the ill-effects on health of many development projects. Hughes and Hunter (1970) suggested a new category of diseases, which they called 'developo-genic', that were analogous to the iatrogenic diseases in medicine but which were caused by the unanticipated consequences of the implementation of development schemes. Such arguments, however, made few dents in the generally held assumptions that developing countries were as yet unformed, infant versions of modern Western societies. By following the same historical path as these societies, and particularly through industrialization, development theorists believed the less-developed countries would become 'developed' in the sense of having high per capita national incomes. Implicit in this theory was the belief that the benefits of growth would 'trickle down' to the poorest sections of society. Although an emphasis on expanding material production was not necessarily inconsistent in practice with the expansion of social services, as Russian experience had shown, most development theorists in the capitalist world believed that the two were incompatible unless accompanied by draconian (and therefore unacceptable) political measures.

However, by the late 1960s and early 1970s there was growing scepticism as to who was benefiting from development (Myrdal *et al.* 1968). In many countries with high rates of economic growth, the rapid rise in per capita income was firmly concentrated in the hands of fairly small numbers, and many groups were worse off than they had been:

> If one examines the 32 individual countries for which data are available, it will be found that the number of 'destitute' people increased in 17 countries in 1963–72 and the number of persons suffering from serious poverty increased in 14 (ODC/ILO 1976).

It was agreed that the 'miracle' of the 'green revolution' (increases in agricultural output based on high-yielding varieties of cereals) had actually led to no improvement in the productivity and income of poor farmers, but rather to increasing marginalization of subsistence farmers.

Changing attitudes towards inequalities between social groups were not limited to developing countries. From the early 1960s onwards, the capitalist developed world was 'rediscovering' poverty (Harrington 1962; Abel-Smith and Townsend 1970), and the debate engendered by revelations of grave differences between social classes led to a spate of rethinking about social policies, stimulating new policy initiatives such as positive discrimination (Evetts 1970). Such ideas filtered into the health field through writings such as those of Bryant (1977) and Navarro (1977) on social injustice and health, and in the 1970s the inequalities of health experience between social groups in both developed and less-developed countries gained more attention.

Inequalities between groups formed the basis for some criticisms of the practice of defining development mainly in terms of national income. Seers (1977), for example, argued that it was more pertinent to look at unemployment, inequality and poverty. If they had all worsened, then even if gross national product were rising, this was hardly a successful measure of development. He disagreed with earlier schools of economists who had always argued that in order to have growth, inequality was necessary: that rapid development demanded a high level of investment which could only come from the profits and savings of the rich, and that if these were squandered on better services for the poor, development would not occur. In the early 1970s experiences of poor countries like China and Sri Lanka, as well as middle-income countries such as Cuba and Costa Rica, suggested that it was possible to have high rates of growth *and* to redistribute some of the benefits to the poor, thus improving their relative position (Streeten 1981). Growth and redistribution were not incompatible even within a capitalist system.

Inequalities between groups broadened to a concern with inequalities between countries. Development theories that assumed the context of a capitalist or mixed economy operating in a capitalist internationalist system led some critics to argue that underdevelopment could not be seen outside the historical context of a world economy dominated by capitalism (Frank 1967; Baran 1973). The reasons for continuing underdevelopment lay not within the underdeveloped countries themselves but in their weak position within a capitalist system dominated by the industrialized powers. Thus developing countries had special problems largely engendered by those nations whose industrialization had taken place at their expense. Many writers, including non-Marxists, accepted Baran's emphasis on the constraints on national development imposed by the international economic system. These writers made up the 'dependency' school.

Dependency was also seen as a technological and intellectual problem. The case in relation to health was argued succinctly by Navarro (1974) and Banerji (1974), who showed the negative effects in Latin America and India, respectively, of using the developed world's concept of health services and medical care. The inappropriateness of Western medical ideology and practice became a central issue in changing ideas about health.

It was perhaps the International Labour Office (ILO) World Employment Conference in 1976 that most clearly rejected past strategies for development and identified a new priority based on the eradication of poverty, the provision of basic needs and productive employment for the whole population. The ILO conference turned from a narrow focus on jobs to *basic needs*, with minimum targets set for food consumption, clothing, housing and the provision of essential services in the areas of water, sanitation education, health and public transport (ODC/ILO 1976).

The shift in thinking expressed at the conference had emerged over several years, at least partly as a result of experience in a number of countries (Jolly 1976). It was not confined to the ILO but mirrored by many other institutions. It became more acceptable to see health as integral to development. The World Bank, for example, which had sometimes financed health components of development projects in various sectors, adopted a formal policy towards health in 1974, although it was only in 1980 that it began direct lending for health programmes (World Bank 1980).

By tracing briefly the changing emphasis in development theories it is possible to see how attitudes to health also changed, and how it began to be seen as part of an integrated package that would help conquer underdevelopment (ODI 1979). The overwhelming concern in the health sector was with unequal access to, and availability of, health services. Rural populations were being grossly neglected in favour of urban populations, and in urban areas the poor were neglected in favour of the better-off. Changing ideas helped to lay the basis for the PHC approach.

Concern about population growth

During the 1960s one of the common explanations for poor countries' slow rates of development was that economic growth was being dissipated because it had to be divided among ever more people. The growth in population was seen by many as a fundamental brake on development. The concern of the developed world, however, was not neutral: it stemmed from the argument that the world's resources were finite, and focused on the one hand on pollution and misuse of existing resources, and on the other on increasing consumption demands. This last was made painfully clear to the rich countries by a shift in power towards the oil producers in the early 1970s. But concern was not only, or even primarily, about limited resources and growing populations; it was also about political security. In his presidential address to the World Bank, Robert McNamara (1979) was quite explicit about the dangers of uncontrolled population growth, suggesting it could lead to high levels of poverty, stress and overcrowding which would threaten social and military stability.

However, the developing world's view of the population 'explosion' did not always coincide with the developed world's view. At the United Nations' World Population Conference in Bucharest in 1974 the Chinese Under-Minister of Health said: 'Is it because of overpopulation that unemployment and poverty exist today? No, it is due to the exploitation, aggression and plunder of the Super Powers' (*The Guardian*, 22 August 1974). At the same conference the Brazilian delegates were even more explicit: they argued that they needed an expanded population because all the great powers had large populations (Bunyard 1974).

Population growth has been a subject of considerable controversy since before Malthus, but until the 1960s birth control was considered a private affair, even in the developed world, and certainly not a concern of the state (Jeger 1962). It was no accident that this changed rapidly with the introduction of the oral contraceptive – officially sanctioned in the industrialized world in 1960, having been tested in the Third World (Vaughan 1970). The oral contraceptive seemed at first sight to be a technological breakthrough which would revolutionize control over fertility. In 1966 the World Health Organization (WHO) reversed a 1952 decision to refuse to undertake a population programme by cautiously agreeing to give technical advice on the development of family planning activities, but only on request (Cox and Jacobson 1973). In 1969 the United Nations Fund for Population Activities was established, and by the 1970s well over US $300 million per year was being spent on population activities by international, national and private sources, three-quarters of which went into family planning (Berelson *et al.* 1980).

Enthusiasm for birth control services as a panacea for population growth was tempered by the pressures exercised to make people use the new technologies, especially in India, raising ethical and moral questions (Banerji 1974), and also by unexpected resistance to contraceptive measures (Bicknell and Walsh 1976). This was paralleled by the trend against vertical services, and by the end of the 1970s it was increasingly accepted (although not everywhere) that family planning (or family spacing) should be integrated into maternal and child health (MCH) services.

However, greater understanding of the issues has not diminished the argument in favour of limiting population growth through birth control. Most developing and developed countries accept that fertility must be controlled if poor countries are to develop:

The real case for an active population policy is simply that, so long as the labour force is growing fast, it is almost impossible to relieve unemployment and poverty since a plentiful supply of labour keeps the wages of the unskilled, apart perhaps from a privileged modern sector, near levels of barest subsistence. Moreover, the growing pressure of population on the budget makes it very difficult to expand educational and other social services (Seers 1977).

Furthermore it has become increasingly clear, although the evidence is scattered, that many Third World women want to control their fertility, and, given methods that are feasible and acceptable to them, are doing so (Population Reports 1984). The emphasis in the 1980s was on integrating family planning into MCH services, not on providing them as a vertical programme, with the focus on family welfare to protect maternal and child morbidity and mortality.

Disillusion with the medical care model

In the mid-1960s Maurice King's (1966) widely disseminated book articulated a different approach to health services, particularly in Africa. The book was the result of a symposium in East Africa, and reflected many people's concern about the inappropriateness of the Western model of medical care being imposed on, or copied by, developing countries. It also reflected a general disillusionment with purely medical solutions. In spite of enormous inputs, many mass disease control programmes were failing for both technical and organizational reasons (Cleaver 1977). There were successes, like the reduction of yaws, the control of malaria in some areas, and later the eradication of smallpox, but the major debilitating or killer diseases – such as tuberculosis, gastro-enteritis and measles – continued to take their toll. Many development projects, such as irrigation schemes or feeding programmes, had had the unintended consequences of actually causing more disease (Taghi Farver and Milton 1973). There were no 'medical' solutions for malnutrition, a major complicating condition in many children's illnesses. The magic bullets capable of reaching and destroying the responsible demons within the body of the patient (Dubos 1959) did not exist. It was clear that other solutions – social, educational, economic and political – had to be sought.

Reaction against mechanistic solutions to illness was one side of the equation. The other was disillusion with hospital-based and hospital-orientated medical services. King (1966) emphasized the importance of looking at the community's needs, arguing that health services and training should be culturally based, and placing the underlying cause of most disease at the level of poverty. In order to increase access to health services the use of medical auxiliaries was strongly advocated and a general attitude, taken up by others later, was that appropriate technologies should be developed. Expensive medical equipment and sophisticated skills did not make sense in countries where foreign exchange was at a premium. It was during the mid-1960s that the idea of *basic health services* (WHO 1973) was developed, advocating the further extension of peripheral health centres and dispensaries – improving access by taking services to where people lived. (It is easy to confuse the basic needs approach as enunciated by the International Labour Office in 1976 (discussed above) and basic health services which emerged as an alternative to centralized hospital services.)

The basic health services policy paved the way for the PHC approach, by recognizing the inappropriateness of hospital care for many of the conditions that were being brought to hospitals, in the absence of alternatives, and by acknowledging that many sick people lived too far away to get to hospital in time for effective treatment. Basic health services, it was argued, had to be not only *available* but also *accessible* and *acceptable* to people. Later a fourth A was added: services had to be *appropriate*.

These ideas from sections of the medical profession were supported by social scientists increasingly 'poaching' on the medical area, and raising doubts about the assumption that disease could be fully accounted for by the medical disease model based on molecular and cellular biology as its basic scientific discipline (Engel 1977). Anthropologists, sociologists and psychologists increasingly showed the importance of other factors.

There were also immense problems of management, side-effects and unintended consequences in the prescription of drugs. Although sulphonamides in the 1930s and antibiotics in the 1940s had greatly increased medical effectiveness in disease treatment, medical intervention with some widely used psychotropic drugs was criticized for their sometimes negative addictive and dependency-creating effects. Illich (1975) argued that medical action or pharmaceutical solutions all too often made illness worse. Criticisms in the developed world were not limited to medical intervention, however. The medical profession's monopoly of knowledge was closely examined; dissatisfaction was being expressed with the private medical systems. Concern about the rising costs of medical treatment added weight to the doubts expressed about health systems in general. All these issues served to raise questions about the medical disease and medical care models, and to shift health care from professional protection. In Britain and the USA the self-care movement grew rapidly in the early 1970s, producing accessible information about health in books such as *Our Bodies Ourselves* (Boston Women's Health Book Collective 1973). It brought the politics of health care into the open.

The issues were, of course, just as relevant to the Third World. The importation of expensive and sophisticated technology and training programmes to deal with relatively rare conditions in developing countries represented a disproportionately high part of the national health budget. Further, it was clear that sick people sought help from a variety of sources, not only Western-trained doctors, and recovered (Kleinman and Sung 1979). The 'witchdoctor' slowly became the less pejorative 'traditional' or 'indigenous' practitioner, and traditional midwives were recognized to be doing useful work in their communities. 'Medical' care increasingly became 'health' care.

Much of the debate that followed centred around the diffusion of technology: how, and why, independent countries retained colonial health infrastructures, and aspired to ideals that were inappropriate to the health situations in their own countries. From India, for example, Banerji (1974) suggested that the colonial inheritance had had deleterious effects on health services. The inappropriateness of selection and training, he suggested, had alienated health workers from the people they served. The costly emigration of newly graduated doctors to the Western developed world was indicative of a professional identification reinforced by inappropriate training, as well as the pull and push of market forces.

The focus on the inappropriateness of aspects of Western-type medical training for developing countries spilled over into other areas. For example, pharmaceuticals came under scrutiny, not only because of the often unscrupulous behaviour of multinational drug companies, but also because of poor prescribing habits, and the plethora of brand-named drugs which added to the costs of many countries' health services (Muller 1982).

While the pattern of thinking about health was moving from medical care to health services and from disease care to health care, what was not really being discussed from within was the notion of community involvement in its own health care. That came from another source, during the 1970s, especially from reports of experiences in China.

Community involvement and self-care

The idea of the Chinese barefoot doctor fired the imagination of the international health establishment. CHWs in various guises had worked closely with health professionals for decades: the idea was not entirely new in the 1970s. What *was* new, however, was the large scale on which CHWs were trained, and in some cases the role they were envisaged to play. In many situations CHWs were seen as a way to extend services to otherwise neglected groups (given the financial and time constraints of training nurses and doctors), and to relieve professionals of routine, rudimentary treatment or preventive actions. In a few situations, however, the role of the CHW was seen much more as political. Here the emphasis was less on service delivery and more on the determinants of health, and the way in which CHWs could rally their communities to tackle these: CHWs were seen as agents of change.

What enthused people about the Chinese system was the active interrelationship between the barefoot doctors and their communities, and the claims of success of mass mobilization against endemic and preventable diseases such as schistosomiasis. Not only were barefoot doctors apparently offering health care to rural populations never before reached by formal health services, but they were accountable to – and controlled by – their own community through the co-operative financial schemes which allowed them to work in the fields part-time, and provide treatment part-time. The first reports by Westerners visiting China were relatively euphoric about the Chinese model, and it was only later that questions about its exportability were raised.

A handful of countries made radical shifts in health policy in the 1950s and 1960s, and by the 1970s were receiving international attention for the resulting improvements in health status. Cuba, which lost one-third of its doctors after the revolution, reconstructed its basic health services, building up a network of polyclinics or health centres, and brought down its infant mortality rate to one substantially lower than that of the rest of Latin America (Huberman and Sweezy 1969). Although using a fairly traditional model for its health service, Cuba instigated a variety of forms of popular community participation, and health workers were expected to spend a relatively large part of their time in community activities (Guttmacher and Danielson 1979). Vietnam (McMichael 1976) and Tanzania (Chagula and Tarimo 1975) also reported imaginative preventive and health care policies utilizing CHWs. In all these countries there was some involvement of the community in health, whether through local organizations or education campaigns (Hall 1978).

The 1970s were fertile years in the exchange of ideas about alternatives in health care, with more emphasis being put on people taking control of their own health and recognizing the positive aspects of self-care. Many of these ideas had grown out of necessity: the Algerians fighting a liberation war found that the people accepted and promoted health measures they had rejected when they had been prescribed by foreign colonialists (Fanon 1965). In the war against the Portuguese colonialist army in Mozambique, Frelimo had almost no medical resources and had to promote ideas of self-sufficiency and self-reliance in health care as in other areas (Walt and Wield 1983).

Aside from these countries fighting for independence, many small-scale voluntary projects run by missionary groups, aid agencies and voluntary organizations had been in existence for a number of years, in a variety of already- or long-independent countries. Many mirrored the principles developed in the community development projects of the 1950s and early 1960s. They all attempted to improve the general living conditions of poor, rural communities with their active participation, by improving skills and encouraging innovation and self-reliance. Multi-purpose workers, who lived in the communities, tried to stimulate community initiative when it was not spontaneous (Holdcroft 1978).

Many non-governmental organizations built on community development ideas and related them to health. By the mid-1970s there were instances of ordinary village people receiving a short training and returning to their own villages to deliver a rudimentary primary care service (Newell 1975). Although such projects often underlined the difference that could be made to a community's health by community participation and mobilization, they also had the negative effect of emphasizing the powerlessness of the community within the larger society intent on preserving the status quo. They were also usually dependent on the voluntary organizations for limited financial support, which was not always sustained.

By the mid-1970s there was also increasing acknowledgement of community resources: traditional midwives were still delivering most babies, mothers and mothers-in-law giving advice. Anthropological studies added to general knowledge and showed that many health actions people took themselves were reasonable. This changing emphasis was accompanied in the industrialized world by the movement in favour of self-care and support networks, and increasing awareness about lifestyle effects on health.

Activities and policies of the international organizations

Two international organizations in particular promoted the PHC approach, WHO and Unicef, the latter initially playing the supporting role to the health professionals. The 1978 public launching of 'Primary Health Care' at Alma Ata as a vehicle for 'Health for All by the Year 2000' was, however, the result of long discussions about policy in both organizations.

Changes in health policy: the World Health Organization

In the early 1970s many people within WHO, or connected with the organization, felt that basic health services were not keeping pace with changing populations, either in quantity or quality. The basic health services concept (see above), which had emerged as an alternative to centralized hospital services in the 1960s, and to earlier vertical disease control programmes, was critically examined by a special working group set up by WHO. This group (WHO 1973) reported that:

> There appears to be widespread dissatisfaction of populations with their health services. ... Such dissatisfaction occurs in the developed as well as in the third world.

The report went on to enumerate the reasons for such dissatisfactions, which included failure of health services to meet people's expectations; inadequate coverage; great differentials in health status within and between countries; rising costs; and a feeling of helplessness on the part of the consumer who feels (rightly or wrongly) that the health services and the personnel within them are progressing along an uncontrollable path of their own which may be satisfying to the health professions, but which is not what is most wanted by the consumer.

The report had two important effects – one conceptual, the other promotional. Conceptually, it laid the basis for the PHC approach. Although it concentrated almost totally on health services and the health sector, it emphasized the need to involve the consumer, to tap local resources, to 'make medicine "belong" to those it should serve' and called for a 'national will' as well as 'international will' for positive health. Promotionally, the report drew attention to WHO's role as 'world health conscience':

It is possible to use WHO not only as a forum to express ideas or dissatisfactions but also as a mechanism which can point to directions in which Member States should go ... as catalytic mechanisms by which those who agree to follow a new path can be assisted.

As part of the search for new solutions to problems in health services, the WHO–Unicef Joint Committee on Health Policy commissioned a study of successful programmes using alternative strategies for providing health care. A number of countries, and many non-governmental organizations, had been experimenting with new ideas in health service delivery. The expansion of health services – through auxiliaries, health centres and involving communities – had begun in a small way in many countries, often by non-governmental missionary groups, but also by governments. By sifting through a great deal of information provided by organizations such as the Christian Medical Commission, and drawing on the health network, it was possible to identify a number of radical approaches to traditional health services which seemed to offer hopeful alternatives. Nine such schemes were described in a book published by WHO in 1975 (Djukanovic and Mach 1975). The same year Newell (1975) covered some of the same programmes, but with more emphasis on the role of communities in health.

In the meantime WHO began to take a much more active role in persuasion and promotion of a particular health message, firmly orchestrated by Halfdan Mahler, who became director-general in 1973. In 1975 he launched the idea of 'Health for All by the Year 2000' as WHO's contribution to the UN's 'New Economic Order', proposing urgent action now to achieve 'in the twenty-five years of a generation what has not hitherto been achieved at all' (Mahler 1975). By this he meant action to achieve 'an acceptable level of health evenly distributed throughout the world's population'. The message was that health had to be considered in the broader context of its contributions to social development. The duty of health professionals was to consider the benefits of all health actions in terms of their social value rather than of their technical excellence. Health was to be used as a lever for social development. 'Health for All by the Year 2000' was endorsed by the World Health Assembly in 1977.

It was in this climate of ideas (and preceded by a number of national and regional meetings on PHC) that the International Conference on Primary Health Care was held at Alma Ata in 1978, sponsored by Unicef and WHO, with a substantial financial contribution from the host country, the Soviet Union. A report on primary health care was prepared and circulated beforehand, and from the meeting, attended by representatives of 134 governments and sixty-seven international organizations, came twenty-two recommendations (WHO/Unicef 1978). The Declaration of Alma Ata outlined the role of PHC in Health for All by the Year 2000:

> A main social target of governments, international organizations and the whole world community in the coming decades should be the attainment by all the peoples of the world by the year 2000 of a level of health that will permit them to lead a socially and economically productive life. Primary health care is the key to attaining this target as part of development in the spirit of social justice (WHO/Unicef 1978).

Community health worker programmes were seen as one of the strategies for PHC. In the Alma Ata document produced after the conference, the rationale behind CHWs was clear:

> For many developing countries, the most realistic solution for attaining total population coverage with essential health care is to employ community health workers who can be trained in a short time to perform specific tasks. They may be required to carry out a wide range of health care activities, or, alternatively, their functions may be restricted to certain aspects of health care. ... In many societies it is advantageous if these health workers come from the community in which they live and are chosen by it, so that they have its support (WHO/Unicef 1978).

The people from the less-developed world who attended the conference (largely ministers of health and their officials) took home with them some of the evangelizing spirit of Alma Ata. Over the next few years a great deal of enthusiasm was expounded at all levels to promote PHC strategies, and to many ministries of health it seemed that the quickest, most visible way of demonstrating their support for PHC was to introduce a CHW programme on a national scale, or to expand small-scale programmes so that they covered larger areas of the country. Those countries that had already introduced CHW programmes (even if not so named) received a fillip of interest, and sometimes even some resource support for training. However, as we shall see in the next chapter, what was meant by a CHW differed from place to place and there was often a large gap between the concept and what happened in practice. Expectations of what CHWs could achieve turned out to be wildly unrealistic.

References

Abel-Smith, B. and Townsend, P. (1970). *The Poor and the Poorest*. Occasional Papers in Social Administration, Bell & Son, London.
Banerji, D. (1974). Social and cultural foundations of health services.systems. *Economic and Political Weekly*, special no., 1333–46.
Baran, P.A. (1973). *The Political Economy of Growth*. Penguin, London.
Basta, S.S. and Churchill, A. (1974). *Iron Deficiency Anaemia and the Productivity of Adult Males in Indonesia*. Staff Working Paper no. 175. World Bank, Washington, DC.
Beenstock, M. (1980). *Health, Immigration and Development*. Gower: Farnborough.
Berelson, B. *et al.* (1980) Population: current status and policy options. *Social Science and Medicine*, 14c, 77–97.
Bicknell, F. and Walsh, D. (1976). Motivation and family planning incentives and disincentives in the delivery system. *Social Science and Medicine*, 10, 579–83.
Boston Women's Health Book Collective (1973). *Our Bodies Ourselves*. Simon and Schuster, New York.
Bryant, J. (1977). Principles of justice as a basis for conceptualizing a health care system. *International Journal of Health Services*, 7, 707–19.
Bunyard, P. (1974). Brazil – the way to dusty death. *The Ecologist*, 4, 83–93.
Chagula, W.K. and Tarimo, E. (1975). Meeting basic needs in Tanzania. In Newell, K. *Health by the People*. WHO, Geneva.
Cleaver, K. (1977). Malaria and the political economy of public health. *International Journal of Health Services*, 7, 557–80.
Cox, R.W. and Jacobson, H.K. (1973). *The Anatomy of Influence*. Yale University Press, New Haven, CT and London.
Djukanovic, V. and Mach, E. (1975). *Alternative Approaches to meeting Basic Health Needs in Developing Countries*. Unicef/WHO, Geneva.
Dubos, R. (1959). *Mirage of Health*. Doubleday, Garden City, NY.
Engel, G.L. (1977). The need for a new medical model: a challenge for biomedicine. *Science*, 196, 129–36.
Evetts, J. (1970). Equality of education opportunity: the recent history of a concept. *British Journal of Sociology*, 21, 425–30.
Fanon, F. (1965). *A Dying Colonialism*. Penguin, Harmondsworth.
Frank, A.G. (1967). *Capitalism and Underdevelopment in Latin America*. Monthly Review Press, New York.
Grosse, R.N. and Harkavy, O. (1980). The role of health in development. *Social Science and Medicine*, 14c, 165–9.
Guttmacher, S. and Danielson, R. (1979). Changes in Cuban health care: an argument against technological pessimism. *Social Science and Medicine*, 13c, 87–96.
Hall, B.L. (1978). Mtu Ni Afya – Tanzania's health campaign. *Information Bulletin*, 9. Clearing House on Development Communications, Washington, DC.
Harrington, M. (1962). *The Other America*. Penguin, London.
Holdcroft, L. (1978). *The Rise and Fall of Community Development in Developing Countries 1950–1965*. Rural development paper, Michigan State University.
Huberman, L. and Sweezy, P. (1969). *Socialism in Cuba*. Modern Reader Paperbacks, New York.
Hughes, C. and Hunter, J. (1970). Disease and 'development' in Africa. *Social Science and Medicine*, 3, 443–93.

Illich, I. (1975). *Medical Nemesis: The Exploration of Health.* Calder and Boyars, London.

Jeger, L. (1962). The politics of family planning. *Political Quarterly* 33, 48–58.

Jolly, R. (1976). The world employment conference: the environment of basic needs. *Overseas Development Institute Review*, 10, 31–44.

King, M. (1966). *Medical Care in Developing Countries.* Oxford University Press, Oxford.

Kleinman, A. and Sung, L.G. (1979). Why do indigenous practitioners successfully heal? *Social Science and Medicine*, 13b, 7–26.

McMichael, J.K. (1976). *Health in the Third World: Studies from Vietnam.* Spokesman Books, Nottingham.

McNamara, R. (1979). Address to the governors of the World Bank, Belgrade, 2 October.

Mahler, H. (1975). Health for all by the year 2000. *WHO Chronicle*, 29, 457–61.

Muller, M. (1982). *The Health of Nations.* Faber and Faber, London.

Myrdal, G. *et al.* (1968). *Asian Drama.* Pantheon, New York.

Navarro, V. (1974). The underdevelopment of health and the health of underdevelopment: an analysis of the distribution of human health resources in Latin America. *International Journal of Health Services*, 4, 5–27.

Navarro, V. (1977). Justice, social policy and the public's health. *Medical Care*, XV, 363–70.

Newell, K. (1975). *Health by the People.* WHO, Geneva.

ODC/ILO (1976). *Employment, Growth and Basic Needs: A One-World Problem.* Overseas Development Council and International Labour Office, New York.

ODI (1979). *Integrated Rural Development.* Briefing paper 4. Overseas Development Institute, London.

Population Reports (1984). *Healthier Mothers and Children through Family Planning.* Series J, 27, 669–78.

Seers, D. (1977). The meaning of development. *International Development Review*, XI, 2, 2–7.

Streeten, P. (1981). *First Things First: Meeting Basic Human Needs in Developing Countries.* World Bank, Washington, DC.

Taghi Farver, M. and Milton, J. (eds) (1973). *The Careless Technology.* Tom Stacey, London.

Vaughan, P. (1970). *The Pill on Trial.* Penguin, Harmondsworth.

Walt, G. and Wield, D. (1983). *Health Policies in Mozambique.* Open University, Milton Keynes.

Weisbrod, B.A. *et al.* (1974). Disease and economic development: the impact of parasitic diseases in St Lucia. *International Journal of Social Economics*, 1, 1, 111–17.

WHO (1973). *Organizational Study on Methods of Promoting the Development of Basic Health Services.* Official records of the WHO, no. 206, Geneva.

WHO/Unicef (1978). *Alma Ata 1978: Primary Health Care.* Health for All Series, 1, Geneva.

World Bank (1980). *Health Sector Policy Paper.* World Bank, Washington, DC.

2 | Who are the community health workers?

Promotion of primary health care (PHC) after Alma Ata led many countries to plan for national community health worker (CHW) programmes. Some had already done this, of course: Botswana's pilot scheme started in 1969 and had been accepted as a national programme in 1973; Jamaica introduced an experimental project in 1967, which was adopted as a national programme by the Ministry of Health five years later. But most countries only started formulating CHW programmes on a large scale at the end of the 1970s. Many countries gave their CHWs special names, such as community health aides (Jamaica), or family welfare educators (Botswana), or village health guides (India). The term *community health worker* was only generally used in the 1980s. Before that it was common to talk of village health workers, primary health workers or even auxiliary workers. Table 1 outlines selected national CHW programmes.

What did countries base their CHW plans on? There were two types of model which by then had received a great deal of publicity: national programmes such as the Chinese barefoot doctor scheme; and small-scale, usually non-governmental projects employing CHWs. The style and ideology of these models differed, but they shared two common aims: to extend health care to underserved populations; and to involve members of the community in their programmes. They could be distinguished by their emphasis on the role of CHWs: as extenders of health care or as catalysts in a development process. Both these roles influenced the programmes of the late 1970s and 1980s and, in many instances, led to unrealistic expectations of CHWs and what they could achieve. Insufficient consideration was given to the extent to which experiences from other programmes could be replicated elsewhere. What went wrong?

Table I Selected national community health worker programmes.

Country	Programme started[1]	CHW name	No. of CHWs trained[2]	Paid/Vol	Male/Female dominated	Source (see index for additional sources)
Botswana	1973	Family welfare educator	609 (1987)	Govt salary	Female	Chapter 7
Burma	1978	Community health worker	19,000 (1983)	Unpaid	90% male	Chauls (1982–3)
		Auxiliary nurse		allowance	Female	
China	1968	Barefoot doctor (1984 became rural doctor)	643,000	Fee-for-service or community pay salary	26% female	Berman et al. (1987) Hsaio (1984)
		Rural health aides	650,000			
Colombia	1969	Health promoter	5,000	Govt salary	Female	Chapter 8
Ethiopia	1978	Community health agent	4,218 (1984)	Community payment	Male	Meche et al. (1984)
India	1977	Village health guide	390,700	Govt honorarium	Male-dominated	Maru (1983) WHO (1987)
Indonesia	1976–7	Nutrition leaders Village health development workers	1,000,000	Volunteers	Female	Berman et al. (1987) WHO (1987)
Jamaica	1972	Community health aides	1,200	Govt salary	Female	Berman et al. (1987) WHO (1987) Cumper and Vaughan (1985) Scholl (1985)
Nicaragua	1981	Brigadistas	41,000	Volunteers	Female	Frieden and Garfield (1987)
Peru	1940s	Health promoters	5,000	Volunteers	Male	Enge et al. (1984)
Sri Lanka	1976	Health volunteers	100,000	Volunteers	Female	Chapter 9
Tanzania	1960s	Village medical helpers/ Community health workers	2,000	Volunteers	Male	Heggenhougen et al. (1987)
Thailand	1977	Village health volunteers Village health communicators	50,000 500,000	Volunteers	Both male and female	Berman et al. (1987) Hongvivatana et al. (1987)
Zambia	1981	Village health workers	4,000 (1986)	Volunteers	Male	Osborne (1983) Twumasi and Freund (1985)

[1] National programmes are often preceded by a pilot or project in a limited area, or take over a number of non-governmental projects which may have run for many years.
[2] It is often difficult to get reliable information on numbers. Numbers trained may be much higher than numbers actively working.

Community health workers as extenders of health services

Some of the earliest CHW programmes were inspired by reports of health professionals who had trained relatively uneducated assistants, often on the job, to do tasks which had been seen as primarily within the professional domain. For example, many doctors in the colonial service in Africa trained *dressers* to unburden themselves of some of the simple tasks which did not necessarily need a physician's level of competence. Miners and plantation workers were trained as *first aiders* to give primary care to their own closed communities, and in war situations community members were trained to give simple medical care to populations with no access to professionals. Such training was usually short and focused mostly on education and prevention, but sometimes included instruction in drugs, first aid and simple treatments.

Some of the first CHWs were trained to specialize in one specific disease: neonatal tetanus (Berggren 1973), childhood diarrhoeal disease (McCord and Kielman 1978), family planning (Zeighami *et al.* 1977) and malaria (Ruebush *et al.* 1985). In the big vertical programmes of the 1950s and 1960s, when governments and international organizations attempted military-style campaigns to defeat specific diseases (yaws, malaria and smallpox), *volunteer malaria workers* were trained for one-and-a-half days to take blood smears and give treatment (Trenton *et al.* 1985), and *lay injectors* were similarly given rapid instruction on how to inject members of the population (Black 1986).

Workers trained rapidly to deal with a specific purpose were not confined to developing countries: in the United States *health guides* were used to improve links between health services and black communities (Warnecke *et al.* 1975). They were recruited from – and visited – families in their own neighbourhoods, and were effective in increasing the use of public health services. In New York City, a CHW programme trained high-school graduates for six months so that they could follow up and encourage preventive behaviour among hypertensive patients (Richter 1974).

While most of the above examples are of small-scale projects, some countries adopted policies to train different levels of professionals to help extend health services to remote areas. The current Russian *feldsher* programme started in the nineteenth century and trained school leavers to provide care to rural populations (WHO 1974). By the mid-1970s, over thirty countries were training middle-level health workers, variously called medical assistants, medical aids, medex workers and physician assistants (Flahault 1974). These and other auxiliary workers were paid workers in particular technical fields, with less than full qualifications in that field, who assisted and were supervised by professionals (WHO 1979). Many had nursing qualifications and, in cases such as the nurse practitioners of the USA, were upgraded in order to provide more services in areas lacking physicians.

These earliest programmes were indigenous attempts to meet local needs:

to train relatively large numbers of health workers quickly and inexpensively to care for communities otherwise badly served by health services. They all faced similar difficulties in financing such policies, in selecting the right people as CHWs, and in keeping them working effectively in isolated situations. Many of those trained deserted their posts for other – often urban – areas, where their prospects for private practice or better-paid employment were greater.

Community health workers as agents of change

For many working in the health field, training community members to provide some rudimentary health care was part of a larger development ideology. Many small-scale projects trained people from the community to provide health care but envisaged such people as catalysts who would help communities understand about ill health and the factors causing it, and help them to change such conditions. Freire's (1972) ideas of empowering communities through an educational process, for example, had a powerful effect on many working in rural development. This concept of 'conscientization', coupled with experiences in non-formal education and community development, led some to argue that CHWs were much more than mere community-based health service deliverers. They were agents of change in a development process, challenging the medical profession's monopoly interest in health care (Rifkin 1978). In the words of Werner (1981), if a CHW is

> taught a respectable range of skills, if he is encouraged to think, to take initiative and to keep learning on his own, if his judgement is respected, if his limits are determined by what he knows and can do, if his supervision is supportive and educational, the chances are that he will work with energy and dedication, will make a major contribution to his community. ... Thus the village health worker becomes an integral agent of change, not only for health care but for the awakening of his people to their human potential, and ultimately to their human rights.

A number of small programmes trained CHWs to take broad, active roles in education as well as treatment. The Jamkhed project in India, and the Gonoshasthaya Kendra project in Bangladesh both recognized a wider, political role for village women in health promotion in the communities (Chowdhury 1981; Chakravorty 1983). The Chimaltenango project in the Guatemalan highlands trained Cakchiquel Indians to provide, among other things, health care (Behrhorst 1984). In all these projects, charismatic leaders – expatriates or nationalists – played a critical part in terms of commitment and support, and were assisted by external funding. The projects usually covered relatively small populations (ranging from a few thousand to one or two hundred thousand people) in contained areas.

The Chinese barefoot doctor scheme encompassed both roles: barefoot doctors were extenders of health services, but they were also part of a political system which emphasized self-reliance at the local level. The financing of the rural medical programme which included the barefoot doctors, however, was only poorly understood outside China, and what was extracted as conventional wisdom from the scheme was a rather simplistic notion that the rural communes supported their own health workers through surplus agricultural production. The fact that China itself went through several systems of local financing, and by 1984 had introduced an individual fee-for-service private practitioner system in many rural areas (Huang 1988), was certainly not recognized at the time most less-developed countries introduced their national CHW programmes. Nevertheless, as perceived by many in the 1970s, the Chinese barefoot doctor was both a provider of health services and a mobilizer of the community.

This, then, was what faced governments in the late 1970s and early 1980s:

- A number of experiences had demonstrated that it was possible to extend services by training health workers for relatively short periods to undertake preventive and curative tasks. In some cases, especially in small schemes, such workers had helped reduce infant mortality rates as well as improve the position of women in the community.
- There was no clear-cut definition of a CHW: the term had been used to encompass relatively well-educated, secondary-school leavers such as barefoot doctors, *feldshers* and auxiliary nurses – some of whom received several years of training – as well as minimally educated, sometimes illiterate, briefly trained primary health workers, health volunteers, health promoters, and village health workers, among others. The diversity of names was reflected in a considerable variety of tasks these workers performed.

The big question was the extent to which it was possible to emulate such projects and apply them nation-wide and in a great variety of different countries.

The formulation of a global strategy

The World Health Organization (WHO) and Unicef started promoting discussion about CHWs from the mid-1970s. In 1977 WHO produced an experimental manual (WHO 1977) and held a number of international meetings with countries that were training CHWs, in order to exchange information on the strengths and weaknesses of existing CHW programmes. At the first of these meetings, held in Jamaica in 1980, it was clear that the definition of a CHW was extremely broad. The participating countries included as CHWs the categories of people shown in Table 2. It was apparent that there were great differences between these CHWs. Some

Table 2 Different countries' descriptions of community health workers in 1980.

BULGARIA	*feldshers*
HONDURAS	Health guardian/Health representative/Traditional birth attendant
PAPUA NEW GUINEA	Aid post orderly
SUDAN	Community health worker
THAILAND	Village communicators/Village volunteers
IRAN	*Behdasht-yar* (male)
	Behvarz (female)
PHILIPPINES	Multiple community health workers
TURKEY	Malaria surveillance agents/Auxiliary nurse midwives/Male public health nurses
BOTSWANA	Family welfare educators
INDIA	Community health worker
JAMAICA	Community health aide
CHINA	Health aids
	Barefoot doctor
ETHIOPIA	Community health agent

Source: WHO (1980)

were salaried workers, with uniforms and pension rights. Of these some were secondary-school leavers, while others had barely six years of schooling. Training was short, but varied from three months to two years. Others received no salary, but were supported in kind by their communities, or were given a small honorarium. Still others worked without payment. The main shared characteristic was that the majority of workers were from *national* programmes – some more advanced than others – which were part of national plans for their countries. The exception was the Philippines, which reported on multiple primary health care projects sponsored by non-governmental organizations.

By starting a process towards a global definition of a CHW the meaning underwent a subtle change. Where CHWs had encompassed a number of different types and categories of worker, the definition gradually narrowed to mean local people who were not expected to move away from the communities which they served. They were preferably women (because their main targets were women and children), but some programmes were dominated by men. They received a very short training and, unlike other health professionals, were unlikely to have the opportunity to be promoted to higher positions, or to be transferred to another part of the country. Sometimes they were paid, sometimes they were not.

The narrowing of the definition of a CHW was not, however, accompanied by any diminution of expectations of what CHWs could do. Underlying the relatively pragmatic planning of national programmes that went on in ministries of health was a great deal of idealistic expectation: CHWs would not only deliver preventive and curative services, and act as the link between the health sector and the community, they would also be responsive and accountable to their communities – who, in their turn, would support CHWs materially or otherwise. One of the flaws in this conceptualization was that although ministries of health might be able to control the health activities of CHWs and their links with the health services, they had no special expertise in matters of community development, in talking to communities, or in rallying community support for CHWs. Very few ministries of health liaised with ministries of community development in the formulation of CHW policy.

Changing definitions of community health workers

It had been expected that most communities would support their own CHWs if they were *selected by* the community, *resident in* the community and were *from* the community. However, doubts about at least one aspect of these expectations were being raised by the early 1980s. A WHO review of national experience in the use of CHWs left out at least one. It suggested the CHW was

> a person from the community who is trained to function in the community in close relationship with the health care system (Ofosu-Amaah 1983).

A later definition suggested that CHWs

> are generally local inhabitants given a limited amount of training to provide specific basic health and nutrition services to the members of their surrounding communities. They are expected to remain in their home village or neighbourhood and usually only work part-time as health workers. They may be volunteers or receive a salary. They are generally not, however, civil servants or professional employees of the Ministry of Health (Berman *et al.* 1987).

It is notable that neither of these definitions insisted that CHWs should be selected by the community. Although this remained a goal of many CHW schemes, experience has shown that community leaders and health-services personnel have a disproportionate say in the selection of CHWs (Jobert 1985; Mburu and Boerma 1986). Taylor's (1986) vivid profile of a village volunteer, Samchai, in Thailand is mirrored the world over:

> He had hoped that being trained as a health volunteer would give him more opportunities to help the other villagers. He had been disappointed not to have been selected when the *puyaiban* first chose people for training three years ago. It was only to be expected, he supposed, that the *puyaiban* would choose his relatives and friends first. But it made him feel so frustrated to see them all pocketing their *per diems* and stowing away their piles of training manuals unread – knowing that they had neither the time nor the inclination to use their

training properly. What was even worse, the son of the *puyaiban*'s best friend – who had gone for the longer, 15-day training to be a health volunteer – did not even live in the village any more. He had gone off to work in Bangkok ...

Two other aspects of the definition above illustrate the gap between ideals and reality facing most CHW programmes. Any government reluctance at having to allocate extra resources – especially salaries – to a CHW programme, could be justified as an ideological concern about accountability. It was argued that volunteer CHWs demonstrated a level of commitment and service to the community that salaried CHWs did not. Moreover, if the community were paying the CHW, in cash or in kind, community members had some control over what they wanted of their CHW. If CHWs were paid by the government, they would have a dual allegiance to their communities and to the health services (Flahault 1978) which could create conflicts of loyalty (Vaughan 1980; Bender and Perry 1982). It is worth looking at these questions of payment and accountability more closely.

Can community health workers afford to be volunteers?

Whether CHWs ought to be volunteers, supported in kind by the community, or paid through community or government funds, has been much debated (de Zoysa and Cole-King 1983). Much of the literature tends to imply that volunteers are the ideal to which most CHW schemes aspire, and assumes that there is sufficient goodwill and personal security to allow relatively poor villagers to conduct voluntary social service (Miles 1985).

It seems the reality is rather different. Most national programmes pay their CHWs either a salary or an honorarium. Almost no examples exist of sustained community financing of CHWs (Gray 1986), and even non-governmental organizations tend to find ways of rewarding their CHWs. Payment is not always direct: some schemes, for example, allow their CHWs and families to receive free health services where they would usually have to pay. And while there are some large-scale programmes where CHWs work on a completely voluntary basis, attrition rates are high (Mburu and Boerma 1986), or the few enthusiastic and reliable volunteers are overloaded with tasks from other agencies and sectors (Heaver 1984).

Why do people volunteer? Studies from industrialized countries such as Britain, where over one-quarter of people over sixteen years do some voluntary work, suggest that there are three basic reasons: reciprocity (helping those who have helped them); beneficence (from a sense of duty and compassion in response to others' needs); and solidarity (feeling some fraternity with others).

While volunteers aim to help or benefit others (or the environment or community) there is an assumed benefit to themselves. Self-interest in voluntarism may be enlightened and motivated by the values mentioned above, or even by a 'consciousness of sin', as was said of the nineteenth-century middle-class in Britain (Pinker 1979). This suggests that the crucial ingredients in volunteering are money and time: a secure economic and social life makes voluntarism possible, even attractive, and may give volunteers a satisfaction they do not get from paid work (Sheard 1986). In both developing and developed countries the men and women who are involved in voluntary organizations usually volunteer their energies from a relatively secure base.

Where does this leave CHW schemes in less-developed countries? Women are in general heavily burdened with daily tasks, with survival or subsistence, particularly poor urban and rural women. There is little time for voluntary work, although there may be considerable reciprocity between neighbours or families at certain times. Religion may play an important part. Among Christians charity is a virtue. In Buddhism voluntarism is a particularly positive value. Another motivating force for volunteering time and labour may be cultural respect for, and compliance with, authority. Status considerations may also be important in motivating volunteers: they are in contact with health professionals such as doctors, nurses and midwives, who usually hold important positions in the community.

The strength of the desire for employment among volunteers is notable, however. In Sri Lanka health volunteers are mainly young, well-educated women who have few job opportunities. When asked, the majority say they volunteer in order to give service, but also that they hope that voluntary work will lead to future employment (Perera and Perera 1985). Job-seeking motivation in voluntarism has been noted in CHW schemes in Nigeria (Adeniyi and Olaseha 1987), Zambia (Harnmeijer 1989) and India (Agarwal 1979; Jaju 1983) where CHWs are paid a small honorarium.

Although in some countries – both developed and developing – volunteers are perceived by policy-makers as a stopgap, or as an alternative to government expenditure, there are exceptions. An ideological religious or political national framework may make a commitment to voluntarism quite widespread. Chauls (1982–3) argues that volunteers in Burma work because the CHWs see themselves as the locus of power in the community which exercises its control through the decentralized power of the Village People's Council.

Voluntary community participation exists in a number of countries – for example, in Cuba, through Committees of the Defence of the Revolution. However, voluntarism organized by the state is inherently contradictory in most societies, although the state may help support relatively autonomous voluntary organizations.

Are salaried community health workers civil servants?

The second question relates to the position of CHWs *vis-à-vis* ministries of health. If those definitions that suggest CHWs are not civil servants or employed by ministries of health were strictly applied, they would exclude many existing CHW schemes. In many countries it is the ministry of health that pays the CHW salary or honorarium, even if this is through another agency (the district council in Zimbabwe, for example). Inasmuch as ministries have the power to withdraw financial support, it could be argued these CHWs are employees or even civil servants, although many of the normal rights of government employees – such as a pension – are often absent. Also, CHWs cannot usually be transferred to another community. What is clear is that in many countries CHWs identify closely with the ministry of health, and the organizational structure of the ministry.

If it is not the ministry of health which pays for the CHW programme, who does? The government of India has had to give a direct grant to the state governments for the CHW honorarium to ensure continuance of the programme, since most states denied it budget priority. Many rural communities are too poor to sustain regular payments to CHWs and, as we have said, the hopes that the Chinese barefoot doctor-commune model could be exported to other countries have been questioned. In the harsh financial realities of the 1980s, many countries tried to extract themselves from being responsible for paying the CHW schemes (Cumper and Vaughan 1985), but passing on the burden for payment to communities was not successful. The problems of the financing of CHW programmes are discussed more fully in Chapter 5.

Idealistic expectations? Rhetoric versus reality

The notion of the CHW in a national programme being an agent of change (not only of individual but also of collective behaviour) was both unrealistic and highly idealistic. By the 1980s a few dissenting opinions were being expressed (Williams and Satato 1980; Werner 1981; Heggenhougen 1984; Jobert 1985; Stark 1985; Cham et al. 1987), but it was striking how little notice had been taken of the extent to which the state and the ministry of health within it would affect policies on CHW programmes, or of how structural conflict, inequality, class or professional dissonance would affect the day-to-day work of the CHW.

Focusing narrowly, most CHW literature ignores the structural distribution of wealth and power, or how health policies entrench patterns of resource distribution, or who gets what services. Yet the context within which CHWs work is all-important. A comparison of health policy development in India and China, for example, shows clearly that the policy of training barefoot doctors was an indigenous idea, and fitted into the organizational structures of rural China. In India the policy to train CHWs was imported, and CHWs were dropped into an administrative vacuum (Chen 1987). Jobert (1985) goes further to suggest that the evolution of the CHW programme in India is an example of the contradictions of populist policies, where resources get diverted and reforms are delayed by the actions of the dominant political and bureaucratic groups.

Because the structural context was not considered in the development of the CHW programme in India, health planners failed to appreciate how great an impact the high rate of unemployment in Indian villages would have on the selection process (Agarwal 1979), resulting in males rather than females being selected as CHWs.

At the opposite extreme, there are documented cases of CHWs being killed or disappearing in repressive and oppressive states (Heggenhougen 1984; Stark 1985). Even where the state is not blatantly repressive, however, there are examples of conflict leading to the murder of CHWs. Chowdhury (1981) describes the death of a CHW in Bangladesh who had begun to expose corrupt practices in a village where free government medicine was being peddled at high profit. In a South African example of a CHW scheme that failed to reach its participatory objectives, those involved asked whether there was any chance of success in a politically, economically and socially oppressive country (Hammond and Buch 1984).

A few case studies have illustrated the kinds of conflict that occur at local levels, affecting the CHWs' work if not putting their lives at risk. Williams and Satato (1980) showed how a PHC programme in Indonesia started enthusiastically training two types of voluntary village health worker, and raising money to provide a rudimentary service at village level. Problems arose when the traditional village authority was challenged (in a small way) by the health committee, and because traditional social relationships – between men and women and between those with land and those without – did not change. The latter in both groups were excluded from all decision-making and planning. Furthermore, the health cadres were co-opted into maintaining 'law and order' by agreeing to join the home guard, a village-level paramilitary organization which was ambivalently regarded by the villagers. Other limitations were put on the project's success by lack of interest and support at regional level.

Several examples from India emphasize the strains upon CHWs who are faced with caste as well as social class differentiations:

> The wealthier families prefer to call the dai to attend deliveries when there are difficulties. ... They do not want to mix with the low-caste women and prefer to treat the dai and health worker as their personal hand-maiden rather than as professionals dispensing a meaningful service (Dyal Chand and Soni 1987).

One study in Madhya Pradesh concluded that the prevailing network of linkages increased and strengthened the old network of the elite, absorbing and distorting the CHW programme:

> The poor who were the supposed beneficiaries had no say in either the decision making or the running of the programme (Quadeer 1985).

Another PHC project, just outside Bombay, which had run for over ten years and successfully trained CHWs, had to close down because of local opposition:

Despite the fact that the poor and even some of the leaders accepted the project services the local power structure dominated by the richer and more powerful leaders joined hands with the government health services in open hostility and demanded that the project leave the area, handing its assets over to them. Their object was achieved after threats and a show of open violence to the project staff (Antia 1985).

In other countries similar tensions have been reported. Twumasi and Freund (1985) describe a CHW in Zambia in conflict with the established local political leaders. Sources of tension revolved around accusations of favouritism in providing services, and overstepping of authority in trying to set up village health committees. The high visibility of the CHW was also regarded negatively by the local politicians.

These conflicts pertain to CHW programmes in particular settings. They underline the importance of considering the political and economic context within which CHWs work. The ideology of the state, and the extent to which it exercises its power through repression or tolerance, will affect the way in which local institutions interact with their own communities. The power relations, of both class and gender, of the wider society are likely to be reflected in what happens at the local level.

Thus, when looking at the way the community health concept developed over the decade of the 1980s, several assumptions have had to be challenged. First, it is clear that, in most national programmes, CHWs are not selected by the communities from which they come: it is the community leaders and the health professionals who ultimately choose the CHWs. There is seldom any democratic process of choice. Second, although it is possible for CHWs to be taken on as volunteers, and not be paid for their services, large-scale volunteer programmes have enormous problems of attrition and may not be cost-efficient. In many national programmes, CHWs not only receive a salary but are, to all intents and purposes, civil servants. They usually identify strongly with the ministry of health. And finally, CHWs in national programmes are not usually able to play the role of change agents: there are too many constraints on them to do this. Instead they act largely as extenders of health services at the periphery. In this sense, they have been highly successful over the last two decades, assisting in an unprecedented expansion of health services to previously neglected areas.

In Part II we will look in more detail at three specific issues relating to CHWs: their tasks and skills; the links between CHWs, the health system and the community; and finally, the problems related to sustaining CHW programmes.

References

Adeniyi, J. and Olaseha, I. (1987). Toward a conflict resolution of multiple perceptions on post-training utilization of VHWs. *Hygie*, 6, 1, 24–8.

Agarwal, A. (1979). Barefoot doctors: symptom not cure. *Nature*, 280, 716–18.

Antia, N. (1985). An alternative strategy for health care? The Mandwa project. *Economic and Political Weekly*, 20, 51/52, 2257–60.

Behrhorst, C. (1984). Health in the Guatemalan highlands. *World Health Forum*, 5, 4, 364–72.

Bender, D. and Perry, H. (1982). The village health worker as a boundary role: caught between two cultures. Paper presented at the 10th International Sociological Association World Congress, Mexico City, August.

Berggren, W.L. (1973). Control of neonatal tetanus in Haiti through the utilization of medical auxiliaries. *Bulletin PAHO*, 8, 1, 24–9.

Berman, P., Gwatkin, D., Burger, S. (1987). Community-based health workers: head start or false start towards health for all? *Social Science and Medicine*, 25, 5, 443–59.

Black, M. (1986). *The Children and the Nations.* Unicef, New York.

Chakravorty, U.N. (1983). A health project that works – progress in Jamkhed. *World Health Forum*, 4, 1, 38–40.

Cham, K. et al. (1987). Social organization and political factionalism: PHC in The Gambia. *Health Policy and Planning*, 2, 3, 214–26.

Chauls, D. (1982–3). Volunteers who work: the community health care project in Burma. *International Quarterly of Community Health Education*, 3.3, 249–66.

Chen, L. (1987). Coping with economic crisis: policy development in China and India. *Health Policy and Planning*, 2, 2, 138–49.

Chowdhury, Z. (1981). The good health worker will inevitably become a political figure. *World Health Forum*, 2, 1, 55–7.

Cumper, G. and Vaughan, J. (1985). Community health aides at the crossroads. *World Health Forum*, 6, 4, 365–7.

de Zoysa, I. and Cole-King, S. (1983). Remuneration of the community health workers: what are the options? *World Health Forum*, 4, 2, 125–30.

Dyal Chand, A. and Soni, M. (1987). The Pachod health programme. In Fernandez, W. and Tandon, R., *Experiments in research as a process of liberation.* Indian Social Institute, New Delhi.

Enge, K. et al. (1984). *Evaluation: Health Promoter Programs*, Ministry of Health, Lima. Management Sciences for Health, Boston, USA.

Flahault, D. (1974). Purposes of the conference on the medical assistant. In Pitcairn, D.M. and Flahault, D. (eds), *The Medical Assistant: An Intermediate Level of Health Care Personnel.* Public health papers, 60. WHO, Geneva.

Flahault, D. (1978). The relationship between community health workers, the health services and the community. *WHO Chronicle* 32, 149–53.

Freire, P. (1972). *Pedagogy of the Oppressed.* Penguin, London.

Frieden, T. and Garfield, R. (1987). Popular participation in health in Nicaragua. *Health Policy and Planning*, 2, 2, 162–70.

Gray, C. (1986). State-sponsored primary health care in Africa: the recurrent cost of performing miracles. *Social Science and Medicine*, 22, 3, 361–8.

Hammond, M. and Buch, E. (1984). Community health workers in Mhala, Gazankula: perversion of a progressive concept? Paper no. 201 presented at 2nd Carnegie Inquiry into Poverty and Development, 13–19 April, Cape Town.

Harnmeijer, J.W. (1989). Personal communication of an unpublished study undertaken in Zambia, 1986.

Heaver, R. (1984). *Adapting the Training and Visit System for Family Planning, Health and Nutrition Programmes*. Staff working paper no. 662, World Bank, Washington, DC.

Heggenhougen, K. (1984). Will primary health care efforts be allowed to succeed? *Social Science and Medicine* 19, 3, 217–24.

Heggenhougen, K. *et al.* (1987). *Community Health Workers: the Tanzanian Experience*. Oxford University Press, Oxford.

Hongvivatana, T. *et al.* (1987). *A Study of Alternatives to the PHC Volunteer and Community Organization Strategy. A Final Report*. Centre for Health Policy Studies, Mahidol University, Thailand.

Hsaio, W. (1984). Transformation of health care in China. *New England Journal of Medicine*, 310, 14, 932–6.

Huang, S.M. (1988). Transforming China's collective health care system: a village study. *Social Science and Medicine*, 27, 9, 879–88.

Jaju, V. (1983). Role of the village health worker – a glorified image. In Jayarao, K.S. and Patel, A.J. (eds), *Under the Lens*. Medico Friend Circle, New Delhi.

Jobert, B. (1985). Populism and health policy: the case of community health volunteers in India. *Social Science and Medicine*, 20, 1, 1–28.

Maru, R. (1983). The community health volunteer scheme in India – an evaluation. *Social Science and Medicine*, 17, 19, 1477–83.

Mburu, F. and Boerma, T. (1986). *The State of MCH/EPI in Eastern and Western Provinces*. Field visit report, Unicef, Lusaka, Zambia.

McCord, C. and Kielman, A. (1978). Successful programmes for paraprofessionals treating childhood diarrhoea and pneumonia. *Tropical Doctor*, 8, 4, 220–5.

Meche, H., Dibeya, T. and Bennett, J. (1984). The training and use of community health agents in Ethiopia. *Ethiopian Journal of Health Development*, 1, 1, 31–40.

Miles, M. (1985). Commentary on Jobert. *Social Science and Medicine*, 20, 1, 27.

Ofosu-Amaah, V. (1983). *National Experience in the Use of Community Health Workers: A Review of Current Issues and Problems*. Offset Publications 71. WHO, Geneva.

Osborne, C. (1983). Community health workers in Zambia. Unpublished report. PHC Secretariat, Ministry of Health, Government of Zambia.

Perera, P.D.A. and Perera, M. (1985). *Study of JOICFP Volunteers of the Ministry of Health*. Marga Institute, Colombo.

Pinker, R. (1979). *The Idea of Welfare*. Heinemann, London.

Quadeer, I. (1985). Social dynamics of health care: the CHW scheme in Shahdol District. *Socialist Health Review*, September, 74–83.

Richter, R. (1974). The community health worker: a resource for improved health care delivery. *American Journal of Public Health*, 64, 11, 1056–61.

Rifkin, S. (1978). Politics of barefoot medicine. *Lancet*, 1, 34.

Ruebush, T.K. *et al.* (1985). Improving malaria detection by volunteer workers. *World Health Forum*, 6, 3, 274–7.

Scholl, E.A. (1985). An assessment of community health workers in Nicaragua. *Social Science and Medicine*, 20, 3, 207–14.

Sheard, J. (1986). *The Politics of Volunteering*. Volunteers Advisory Service: Advance, London.

Stark, R. (1985). Lay workers in primary health care: victims in the process of social transformation. *Social Science and Medicine*, 20, 3, 269–75.

Taylor, D. (1986). *A Tale of Two Villages*. New Internationalist Publications, Oxford.

Trenton, K. *et al.* (1985). Improving malaria detection by volunteer workers. *World Health Forum*, 6, 3, 274–7.

Twumasi, P. and Freund, P. (1985). Local politicization of primary health care as an instrument for development: a case study of community health workers in Zambia. *Social Science and Medicine*, 20, 10, 1073–80.

Vaughan, J. (1980). Barefoot or professional? Community health workers in the Third World. *Journal of Tropical Medicine and Hygiene*, 83, 3–10.

Warnecke, R.B. *et al.* (1975). Contact with health guides and use of health services among Blacks in Buffalo. *Public Health Reports*, 90, 3, 213–22.

Werner, D. (1981). The village health worker – lackey or liberator? *World Health Forum*, 2, 1, 46–54.

WHO (1974). *The Training and Utilization of Feldshers in the USSR*. Public Health Papers, 56. WHO, Geneva.

WHO (1977). *The Primary Health Worker*. WHO, Geneva.

WHO (1979). *Training and Utilization of Auxiliary Personnel for Rural Health Teams in Developing Countries*. Technical Report Series 633. WHO, Geneva.

WHO (1980). Primary health care. The community health worker. Report on a Unicef/WHO interregional study and workshop (Kingston, Jamaica). Unpublished report, PHC/80.2. WHO, Geneva.

WHO (1987). Community health workers: pillars for health for all. Unpublished report of the interregional conference, Yaoundé, Cameroon, 1–5 December 1986. WHO, Geneva.

Williams, G. and Satato (1980). Socio-political constraints on primary health care. *Development Dialogue*, 1, 85–101.

Zeighami, E. *et al.* (1977). The rural health worker as a family planning provider: a village trial in Iran. *Studies in Family Planning*, 8, 7, 184–7.

PART II

Issues

3 | Tasks and skills: what can community health workers do?

There are two conundrums facing community health workers (CHWs). The first is logistic: CHWs are the least well-trained workers in health, yet they are the most isolated and therefore lack the necessary support. The second is conceptual: although many common illnesses are preventable, they are not *easily* preventable.

The main logistic problem is that CHWs are trained for short periods in which they can be taught only a restricted number of skills. Yet, a CHW may often be the only trained health worker in a community and may be asked to cope with a wide variety of problems for many of which he or she cannot provide the answers. Compounding this, CHWs live in relatively remote areas and referrals to higher levels of the health service and supervision by health professionals are difficult to guarantee. Yet in order to sustain the quality of their work, and to reinforce their short training period, they need close supervision and support.

The conceptual problem about the sort of prevention and promotion that CHWs can do is seldom explicitly acknowledged by health professionals. The dominant focus of their work is on individuals within the community, rather than on the environmental setting within which the community lives. CHWs learn preventive skills which draw attention to the potentially unsafe behaviour of individuals (usually mothers), and they are expected to encourage actions to avoid or counteract such behaviour. Thus CHWs spend much of their time advising mothers on, for example, the advantages of breast-feeding, feeding their children particular foods, or giving them sugar-salt solutions during episodes of diarrhoea; or on encouraging families to build and use latrines or home gardens, or to take their children to be immunized. This individualized view of illness is classical of much thinking in health, and while it helps to structure training and the delivery of services its limited perspective deflects attention from important variables in the environment that influence people's behaviour: economic, social and cultural factors. Furthermore, experience in both less-developed and

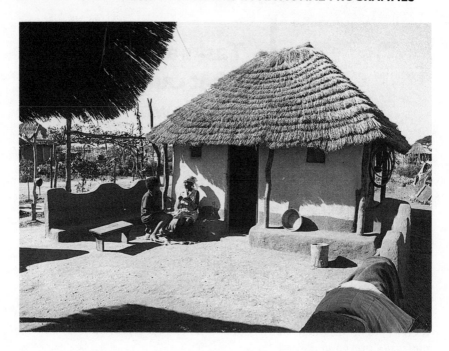

1   *As often the only trained health worker in a community, the CHW needs a wide variety of skills. Here a family welfare educator in Botswana visits a psychiatric patient at home. Photo: WHO by J. Mohr.*

industrialized countries shows that changing individual behaviour is extremely difficult, and that those who do change their ways as a result of receiving information about potential risks are often the groups *least* at risk.

The problems faced by CHWs start with training. Most training is divided into simple curative care, prevention and health education. Although lip-service may be paid to environmental issues, training is usually focused on the classical individualized approach to illness described above. Once CHWs have returned to their relatively remote communities, prior training – even when it was well done – is rapidly undermined by a lack of continuing education or reinforcement through support and supervision. The steady sinking into demoralization because of an inability to help all too often leads to a fall in general activities and a neglect of tasks such as health education. Added to this, even though the CHW may be the only formally trained health worker in the community, people will be accustomed to going to the traditional system for help. An example from Tanzania illustrates this:

> On one of our walks we stopped by a crumbling hut of an elderly couple. The wife was sick, ashen looking, lying on her cot with pain in her right leg, terribly thin and anaemic. No latrine, disorder all around.

The man was busy building a small spirit house where food would be placed to placate the spirits so that his wife would get better. The CHW suggested to the husband that he take his wife to the health centre – but how, when she could not walk? Under the circumstances the CHW could offer no other advice and did not stay to talk about such items as cleanliness, nutrition or latrine construction (Heggenhougen *et al.* 1987).

CHWs, therefore, face terrible dilemmas. They cannot easily change community members' behaviour. They have limited skills and scope for treating illnesses or injuries. And referral is often restricted. How have CHWs in national programmes coped with these difficulties? This often depends on three criteria: what the professional health workers think they ought to do; what CHWs would like to do; and what communities expect CHWs to be able to do.

Community health worker roles

The rationale for training CHWs is based on the knowledge that much ill health is preventable, and on the assumption that most of the problems of ill health faced in a community are fairly common and can be relatively simply treated. Thus CHWs are taught as much about prevention and promotion as about disease.

Although there are differences between countries, the responsibilities CHWs might be given include advising on family planning, antenatal care and safe delivery, and sometimes helping at deliveries – although this is probably quite rare. They may be expected to teach health education on the value of breast-feeding, or on oral rehydration therapy (ORT) and how to make up oral rehydration solutions or use ORT packets. They will have to teach others about diarrhoeal disease, home hygiene – including the building of latrines and home gardens – and various aspects of nutrition. They may also be taught something about the common diseases of the area – such as diarrhoea, respiratory tract infections, malaria and tuberculosis – and how to treat them, as well as how to deal with common accidents such as open wounds. They may have a small selection of drugs to distribute, though these are seldom more than simple analgesics, iron tablets, malaria prophylactics or treatments, and sometimes an antibiotic ointment or other types of antibiotics. It is rare for CHWs in national programmes to be allowed to give injections or vaccinations, unless they do this illegally (there are some reports from India that village health guides buy injections from drug pedlars) or under the supervision of a primary health team either on outreach or at a primary health facility.

A much-debated aspect of the tasks of CHWs is the extent to which they are concerned with prevention or treatment, and whether one takes precedence over the other.

Community health workers as 'mini' doctors

While it is often asserted that being able to treat illness helps CHWs to establish their credibility in a community, some have argued that there are dangers to this, and CHWs may all too easily become 'mini' doctors. In this role they are dangerous in that their claims to cure ills are inflated given the little training they have received, or else distracting because they divert attention from the real problems of health which may be preventable.

Such arguments usually stem from the medical and, occasionally, nursing professions. The medical profession in some countries has been extremely reluctant to allow CHWs access to their more valued treatments and techniques, such as antibiotics or injections. In many communities injections are believed to be more efficacious in treating ill health than other forms of medicine. While some professional concern is based on the fear of injudicious use of injections or medicines – which may have grave long-term consequences if, for example, syringes are not sterile, or antibiotics are used indiscriminately – some also stems from a wish to control other health workers' access to medical techniques. This attitude has been criticized as, for example, in Aitkin's (1986) attack on the stand of some doctors in India, who believe that

> village health workers should not be taught to give injections because they are so susceptible to abuse. I would like to answer that it is those in the medical profession itself who are largely responsible for this abuse ... It is apparently common practice to keep a syringe in a dirty cardboard box, to wipe a needle and rinse a syringe in spirit rather than boil them and to push the needle along one's unwashed index finger while injecting. ... Misuse applies to unnecessarily giving injections as well as to bad techniques ...

Aitkin goes on to point out that doctors are more shielded from repercussions in the event of untoward results from a treatment than are village health workers who live among their patients and have to face them if things go wrong. Very few studies have been done to assess how far CHWs are able to use medicines appropriately. One example from Afghanistan suggested that the benefits of supplying village health workers with penicillin almost certainly exceeded the risks involved, and the antibiotic was not over-prescribed: only 5 per cent of all treatments provided by the village health workers were with penicillin, which had potentially the most risks from misuse of all their available drugs (O'Connor et al. 1980).

The opposite argument, however, is that CHWs will never be able to establish their credibility with the community without being able to offer drugs and to treat common ailments. There is plenty of evidence to show that what community members want in their villages or neighbourhoods is a doctor – or a health worker who can treat illness and accidents. Chandra et al. (1980) found that of all the CHW's tasks, treating minor ailments was the only one used maximally (by 60 per cent of the population), and Sales (1977) argued that in Niger the very availability of drugs – provided by international agencies – created demand for them. The cry by CHWs and communities for regular supplies of medicines is common to many programmes (Heggenhougen *et al.* 1987; Kaseje 1987).

The difficulty is to sustain the balance between treatment and prevention. This also depends on whether the CHW is part- or full-time, is supposed to spend most time visiting people in their homes, or works from a health facility. It seems, however, that where CHWs can provide treatment, especially from a fixed health facility, this is what they and the community prefer, and claims made for the amount of time spent on preventive care should be treated with some scepticism. One small study in Kenya suggested that CHWs actually spent one-third of their time on preventive work and only 1 per cent on curative care (most of their time was spent on travelling and introductions!), but admitted that there were many other sources of medical attention and that CHWs were not sought out as primary care providers (Jacobson *et al.* 1987). A preference for providing curative care was clearly shown among those CHWs who remained active in Tanzania (Heggenhougen *et al.* 1987).

Community health workers as extra pairs of hands

Where CHWs are attached to a health facility there may be a great temptation to spend most time there. In Botswana, where almost a quarter of CHWs work on their own in a health post, community members feel that they should stay there so that they can be consulted when needed: shutting the health post to go on home visits is not seen to be in the community's interests. Where CHWs are part of a larger team of health workers, or work with an enrolled nurse, they are still unlikely to spend a significant amount of time on home visiting. This probably occurs for two reasons.

First, many CHWs express some hesitation about visiting homes to make general preventive visits, and are only marginally less reluctant to do follow-up visits after a patient has been to the health facility. The reasons for this are complex, but include difficulties of possibly seeming to be interfering, differences in social status between the CHW and the family, and the logistic drawbacks of dispersed households, terrain and climate. Second, the nurses in the clinics see the CHWs as useful extra pairs of hands, and are able to devolve what should be their responsibilities upon the CHWs. In busy clinics, CHWs make a useful contribution in sharing the load of patient care, especially the more routine or menial tasks. A study in Thailand reports:

> In essence, most volunteers were simply helping hands for the tambon health workers in routine health activities as child weighing every 3 months, gathering mothers and children and assisting in immunization sessions every 2 months, collecting vital records and other information

relating to maternal and child health and sanitation, and other occasional requests. The active volunteers were doing it routinely for the local health workers, and the health workers knew it (Hongvivatana et al. 1987).

It is understandable why CHWs find such work relatively congenial. They are working side by side with professional staff and derive high status from their position in the health facility. Hours are fixed and regular (professionals working to government regulations), and the conditions are easier than walking around villages house to house. This does not mean that conflict and confusion between the various types of personnel do not exist, as we shall see in the next chapter, but that in many situations working mainly in a health facility is more attractive than home visiting.

Of course, even if CHWs spend most hours in a health facility, much of their time may be spent on preventive activities such as antenatal care, health education, immunization and baby weighing. A time and motion study would be needed to ascertain precisely how the days are parcelled out among the above activities and others such as registration of patients, dispensing of medicines, making up dressings or cleaning the health facility – all activities in which CHWs in Botswana were observed to be involved, as is shown in Chapter 7.

Whether or not the activities in a health facility are preventive or curative, if CHWs spend most of their time in a fixed post they are only attending to those families who go there. Yet there is evidence to suggest that, for a complex series of reasons, it is often the *most in need* who do *not* use health services, so that it is likely that those most at risk in the community will be missed. Whether this should be held as the responsibility of the CHW is another point, however.

Community health workers as educators

In many CHW programmes which rely entirely on volunteers – as in the Sri Lanka example described in Chapter 9 – CHWs have only educative tasks. They are not expected to provide treatment, and if they do it is very circumscribed. The health volunteers in the settlement areas of Sri Lanka can treat malaria, for example. In other programmes CHWs may distribute contraceptives. Thus, although they may help health professionals at clinics their main role is in preventive and promotive health education.

Many doubts have been expressed about the effectiveness of health education alone in changing people's behaviour. It is sometimes argued that only high-status educators may have any real impact on behaviour – which will be influenced by many factors – and that therefore CHWs with health education tasks are likely to be doubly ineffective. Hongvivatana et al. (1987) state that in Thailand:

> In the village socio-cultural settings, [the] educator role is usually reserved for the few who are virtuous, educated (not necessarily in the

sense of formal schooling), senior and well-respected. It is unimaginable for a common villager with 5 days' training to talk health education or to communicate in a deliberate educative sense.

Evidence from CHW programmes is mixed and depends a great deal on community perceptions of what is of value. In some places CHWs have been very successful, for example in rallying communities to attend immunization sessions, so leading to much greater coverage of the population than would have been possible even with health service outreach teams. In Afghanistan such a success was attributed to the value the community placed on injections, resulting directly from the eradication of smallpox (O'Connor *et al.* 1980). It may be less easy to mobilize communities for other activities. For example, it is much more difficult to persuade communities unused to utilizing latrines about their value for health. People may be more easily persuaded for reasons of status, or because they wish to be modern. In the mountains of Lesotho, latrines made of shiny corrugated iron are preferred to latrines built traditionally, of stone, in spite of the fact that the former cannot withstand the high winds of the area while stone dwellings have considerable resistance. But neither latrine is valued highly, and in the unpopulated, dry, hot climate of the mountains latrines probably have a minimal impact on health anyway.

Villagers may also comply with health education activities for hidden motives. Williams (1986) quotes a CHW in Indonesia with responsibilities in nutrition:

We've been doing weighing in our village for five years now, but most mothers still don't understand it very well. What they really want is extra food for their children, not a weighing post. Even those who do come regularly aren't really involved. They hand the child over to the cadre to be weighed like a sack of rice. Then another cadre writes something on the child's growth chart, another gives the child a biscuit or a fried banana – and finally the mother goes home thinking she's done something useful for her child's health. But has she really? I'm not sure.

It may be enough that the mother brings her child to be weighed, since the implication is that if the child's growth is faltering, the health worker can help the mother do something about it. However, research on growth monitoring suggests that this aim is seldom achieved, and that many weighing clinics are often seen as ends in themselves (Gerein 1988). Furthermore, while health education messages are often understood and remembered, they are not always acted upon. Specifically trained CHWs in Bangladesh are able to teach mothers seven points about making sugar-salt solutions to use when children have diarrhoea; they are less successful in getting mothers to use the solution they have made (Chowdhury and Vaughan 1988).

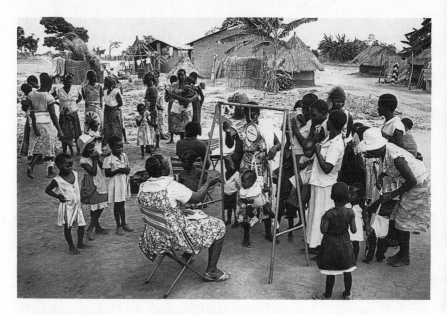

2 *Weighing children is a task CHWs often undertake. At this session in Zimbabwe, mothers also participate. Photo: WHO by Liba Taylor.*

The conceptual and methodological difficulties of assessing the impact of health education are multifarious, but this is not the only aspect that has to be considered in CHW programmes. The other problem is keeping up interest – of both CHW and communities – in a limited range of health education activities. In the village health worker programme in Afghanistan it was noted that the lack of any incentives for these workers to provide preventive or health education services was a major weakness in the scheme, since villagers did not perceive the need for either. The conclusion was that it was doubtful whether village health workers did anything much in the health education field, and that their impact outside their own families was probably negligible (O'Connor *et al.* 1980)

Policy-makers take polar positions on this question. In Sri Lanka the potential educative impact on the family is seen as a positive feature of the health volunteer programme. Thus it is argued that, even if health volunteers drop out of the programme, they still pass on their knowledge to their families, leading to a mass health education effect. However, the conclusion by Hongvivatana (1987) in Thailand is that no more effort should be put into the health communicator programme, where CHW roles are restricted to health education, and that money saved from this short training should be put towards improving the training of health volunteers who are attached to health posts.

Activity levels

Whichever of the above three roles CHWs end up playing – 'mini' doctors, extra pairs of hands, or educators – depends a great deal on the health system to which they are attached. However, it seems from what evidence is available that whatever CHWs do, they are unlikely to be extremely active in carrying out their tasks. Where CHWs work in health facilities their level of activity depends on the leadership and attitude of the head of that facility, and this may differ considerably. In the Botswana study described in Chapter 7, outpatient contacts in health clinics per day per staff member ranged from 5.5 to nearly thirty. CHWs on their own in a health post saw between nine and twenty-two outpatients per day. In Colombia (Chapter 8) – where home visiting is the main activity and clear routines are established – the average number of visits per day was only four. For an average population of 2,100 that the health promoter is meant to cover, each family (assuming about 500 families) could receive between one and two visits per year – assuming 200 working days per year. Making more visits to families at risk would be difficult. Health promoters also spend a substantial proportion of their time on curative services when doing home visits.

Activity levels among volunteers or part-time workers may be especially low, with high percentages of CHWs desisting from any work at all after a time. In Peru, CHWs are part-time volunteers, and the programme which has been in existence in one form or another for over fifty years suffers from high attrition rates. Since the mid-1950s, between 10 and 50 per cent of CHWs have abandoned their work as health promoters. Those who continue tend to have relatively low activity levels, averaging between ten and forty health-related activities per month. Like the Colombian CHWs, most of these activities are related to curative care, and to adults rather than children (Enge et al. 1984). The village health communicator programme in Thailand has also suffered high attrition levels: as of 1986, 62 per cent of CHWs throughout the country had either dropped out completely or else were working only very sporadically. However, attrition rates differed from village to village, and the smaller villages of less than 100 households tended to have more active CHWs. The attrition rates of the village health volunteers (who have more tasks than the village health communicators) were lower, but the quality of their work has been criticized, and in one study only 22 per cent were classified as highly active, 'being enthusiastic and able to plan and conduct PHC work mainly on their own, with minimum interference from the tambon health workers' (Hongvivatana et al. 1987).

Activity levels obviously also depend on the community's perception of the values of the CHW. Few studies have assessed community expectations. Heggenhougen et al. (1987) provide some colourful vignettes of a myriad of CHW relationships with village people. These were gained during stays in villages, and give more detail than is usually available in most descriptions of rural communities. In general, the impression is that villagers are disappointed with the limited range of curative services CHWs are able to provide, and CHWs feel inadequate and frustrated at not being able to meet expectations. An Indian evaluation which claims that community members and health service staff were satisfied with their CHWs (Maru 1983) has to be seen within the constraints of relying on a questionnaire wielded by outside evaluators. CHWs themselves often complain of a lack of support from the community (Sudsukh 1982; Meche *et al*. 1984), and since curative and emergency care are top priorities in most communities, CHWs may not be valued if they are unable to meet such needs. Certainly, experience in Mali and Senegal suggests that failures by communities to find local funds for primary health care (PHC) and CHWs were due to their perception that the benefits were not commensurate with the resources they would have to raise (Gray 1986). In Papua New Guinea many communities were not even aware of what their CHWs did (Frankel 1984).

Given these scenarios it is perhaps not surprising that CHWs in national programmes tend to be extenders of health services, preferring to provide treatment in health facilities or on home visits. For previously underserved or unserved rural populations, they may be filling a real gap. But how good are the services CHWs provide? What is the quality of their care?

Quality of care

To provide good-quality care, CHWs need a solid training, continuing education, a reliable supply of medicines, and regular support and supervision. Unfortunately, these are the very areas which are acknowledged to be weak in many programmes:

> It is alarming to contemplate the number of these lay people whom we have placed in positions of authority; who work without adequate supervision; who distribute advice without knowledge, and who sometimes further their own interests at the expense of the sick (Skeet 1984).

A major problem is that there are few studies that have looked at the technical quality of the service given by CHWs, and the extent to which it is influenced by the above factors. Let us look at each separately.

Training and continuing education

Training differs considerably from country to country, with wide variations in duration and location. Some CHWs are trained in days, others take a third of a year. Some are trained relatively close to their own communities, at the nearest health centre, others many miles away, sometimes in an inappropriate urban setting. Many training programmes have been designed using the classic individualistic concept of prevention of ill health described earlier in this chapter, which affects the kinds of services CHWs then provide in the community. However, although training content is usually relevant to the job CHWs are later expected to do, actual training processes are more problematic. Many of the teachers of CHWs are not full-time trainers, but members of the health team (public health nurses, for example) who teach as an adjunct to their other responsibilities. They have rarely been trained in teaching methods, and usually emulate the way they were themselves taught. Strict classroom discipline and blackboard and chalk didactic methods may be completely inappropriate for relatively poorly educated CHWs. It is seldom that CHW training is based on 'doing', and although most authoritative texts on training emphasize this approach (Abbott and MacMahon 1985), it is not often followed in national programmes. Yet even biological knowledge can be imparted in simple ways. O'Dempsey (1988) describes one example of teaching illiterate CHWs who wanted to know the 'truth' about diseases:

> Starting with the idea 'dog bites man' and scaling down until we reached 'mite bites man' we asked if it was possible that small creatures

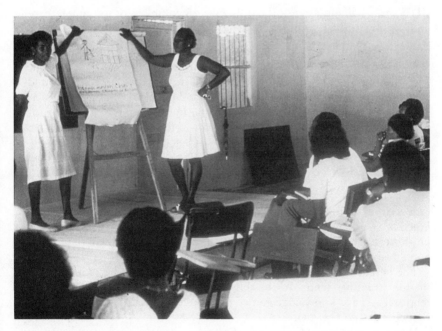

3 Strict classroom discipline: will these student health promoters in Colombia be able to relate what they have learned to the tasks they will later face? Photo: H. Jiménez (Convenio Colombo-Holandés).

exist that might be harmful to man. 'Yes' the CHWs replied 'but we have never seen them'. We then handed around magnifying glasses showing how these made small things appear bigger. Finally we introduced a microscope, and a drop of water, which, everyone agreed, appeared harmless and drinkable to the naked eye, but when viewed under the microscope was seen to be teeming with microorganisms. The CHWs, greatly excited, went home and returned bringing members of the health commitee to see for themselves. Thereafter, we were able to explore various health problems, referring to the 'germ theory' as appropriate.

Common complaints about much CHW training are that it is too theoretical and too complicated, as this description of what a CHW from Thailand thinks about his training graphically illustrates:

The training sessions had made his head swim: there was so much information to digest and it was years since he had sat in a classroom. He had almost forgotten how to read; yet they had given him sixty close-typed training manuals to take away with him. Sixty! He nearly fainted. 'Self-learning modules' they had called them. An apt title, he thought. Because he felt he had been by himself ever since (Taylor 1986).

CHWs in Thailand are not the only ones to complain of too much reading and too much time spent on theory. In Peru it was noted that

during a thirty day course only two days were programmed for teaching outside the classroom. The coordinator of the course said she would have liked to take the students to surrounding health posts and health centers to do practical work, since the Acora Health Center was not large enough for all of the students, but there were not funds for transportation of this sort. Empty spots in the schedule seemed to get filled in with more first aid. The students seemed to prefer more practical, curative topics. One student expressed the opinion that they 'weren't going to cure sick people with talks' (Enge *et al.* 1984).

In Colombia a review of the standard curriculum revealed a possible excess of such subjects as anatomy and physiology, and of theory in general. Practical work was given little emphasis, in spite of the fact that health promoters are expected to spend the great majority of their time making home visits and giving health education.

The extent to which training is followed up by refresher courses or on-the-job training tends to be haphazard. Few CHWs receive regular reinforcement of knowledge gained in initial training courses, much less the chance to learn new materials.

However, training does not have to be formal: much can be learned during supervisory visits by both the supervisor and the CHW, often with the help of manuals. Not only have such manuals been encouraged at the international level by the production of the WHO's (1977) *The Primary Health Worker*, produced as a model for countries to adapt to their particular reality, and by the translation of Werner and Bower's (1982) *Helping Health Workers Learn* into several other languages, but also, during the 1970s and early 1980s, many countries produced their own manuals. As we will see in Chapter 7, for example, Botswana reorientated its curricula for family welfare educators as late as 1987. Whatever shortfalls there are in training programmes, there is no doubt that more time and energy has been put into developing curricula and training manuals than has ever been put into support and supervision.

Support, supervision and supplies

In most national programmes, CHWs are supervised by professional health staff who work from a health facility. Sometimes these are public health nurses, or specialists in community health, but very often they are nurses with clinical duties who give precedence to delivering a service and little attention to supporting CHWs (unless they can be useful in the facility). Supervising CHWs in their own communities may have low priority, especially in countries where transport conditions are poor, vehicles are few, and incentives to supervise are lacking. Even where per diems are allowed they are not always easy to collect:

> The Ministry of Public Health required signatures as proof of travel and also stipulated that the trip must involve a certain minimum number of kilometers. Road conditions to most [village health worker (VHW)] villages were very poor, and adequate transportation for the sanitarian was often unavailable. All these factors combine, and the result was that VHW supervisory visits rarely took place (O'Connor *et al.* 1980).

CHWs are often confused about who is their supervisor. They largely identify the nurses from either their own facility or from the nearest clinic to fill this role. Theoretically, however, the community/public health nurses or family nurse practitioners – who are specialists in community health – are their supervisors. CHWs seldom see their supervisors more than once a month and the visits are often largely a perfunctory glancing over record books. Even where supervisory contacts are relatively frequent, the quality of those contacts may be poor. For example, the Colombian health promoters have a relatively high frequency of contact with their supervisors, either at clinics or when supervisors visit them in their communities. However, the study described in Chapter 8 throws some doubt on the quality of these encounters: most time was taken up with checking the CHW's records and taking an inventory of her equipment, and possibly giving a short didactic talk. If problems were raised they were dealt with cursorily, if indeed the supervisor had the ability to deal with them at all.

Thus supervision was described as theoretical and critical rather than practical and supportive.

If the organization of supervision is problematic, then providing CHWs with regular supplies of medicines is also a weak link in the support chain. Many countries face chronic shortages of drugs at the primary level (even for health facilities), and the isolation of CHWs means that they are often the first not to be restocked. Although traditional remedies and herbs continue to be used in most communities, and health workers have been positively encouraged to prescribe them in some countries (such as China), modern drugs are valued and desired by people even in very remote rural areas. When primary-level health facilities do not have a consistent and regular stock of medicines, their utilization rates fall. In the same way, when CHWs run out of drugs, people lose faith in them and do not consult them. A few countries, for example Thailand, have introduced community-level drug co-operatives. Community members (who are shareholders in the Drug and Medical Products Fund) can then buy drugs from the CHWs who sell them at a small profit. This works well in many villages in Thailand, although not everywhere.

Almost all reviews of CHW programmes have concluded that their weakest points are support, supervision and supplies (Ofosu-Amaah 1983). If this is the case, what are the chances that the quality of work that CHWs do will be good? Assessing quality of care – whether of doctors, nurses or CHWs – is not easy, partly because it is difficult to agree on performance standards, but partly also because it is time-consuming and expensive. (The problems of assessment are discussed in Chapter 6.) The few studies that have tried to assess CHWs' skills have therefore looked at levels of knowledge and relevance of practice, rather than at the technical quality of CHW services.

For example, an evaluation of the Indian national CHW scheme carried out in 1979 found that

> CHWs scored poorly in four areas: conditions requiring referral to higher level health facilities; prevention of disease; emergency treatments; and general preventive, promotive, and curative services. Scores averaged below 30 percent correct responses and in some cases below 20 percent. Very high scores were recorded concerning the use of specific medicines, such as chloroquine, which compose the bulk of the CHWs' purely curative function. In general, for those tasks expected to have a significant long-term impact on health status, CHW knowledge was disappointing (quoted in Berman *et al.* 1986).

Another evaluation, this time of Peruvian CHWs, also looked at knowledge levels. CHWs were relatively well-informed about vaccinations for children (81 per cent could mention at least one vaccination children should have) but not about tetanus toxoid for pregnant mothers, and in general knowledge levels in relation to childbirth and related risks were low.

They did substantially better on diseases: over 80 per cent knew some of the symptoms of tuberculosis, for example (Enge *et al.* 1984). This was possibly indicative of their interests.

A small study in India attempted to assess the work performance of part-time CHWs. Performance indicators were chosen to evaluate the extent to which CHWs were meeting the goals of the programme. These included the percentage of pregnant women who received antenatal care at clinics, the percentage of pregnant women visited at home by CHWs, the number of home deliveries, and so on. From the analysis it appeared that CHWs with less education, less population to cover, and more intense supervision, were the high scorers on work performance. The interesting finding in this study was that CHWs who had higher levels of education performed less well in home visiting because they felt awkward in lower-class households (Bhattacharji *et al.* 1986).

One of the features of this last programme was that it was highly supervised (and was not part of the government CHW scheme). Another well-supervised regional programme – this time in Somalia and supported by Unicef – showed that CHW's levels of knowledge on signs of dehydration, immunization schedules, and pneumonia symptoms and treatment, were high, and more than adequate for their tasks (Government of Somalia/Unicef 1986). Furthermore, it seemed as if CHWs had a clear impact on disease management though not on disease prevention: in the villages with CHWs, 58 per cent of mothers used oral rehydration solutions when their children had diarrhoea, and another 20 per cent used home-made fluids. However, the overall incidence of diarrhoea did not change with the introduction of CHWs (Bentley 1989). This is not surprising given the complicated aetiology of diarrhoeal disease, and it may be unrealistic to expect CHWs to have influenced the incidence of diarrhoea.

A well-supervised programme in Brazil attempted to ascertain the quality of the CHWs' care by estimating two measures: the percentage of third doses of diphtheria, pertussis and tetanus (DPT) inoculation among the population under one year of age, and the percentage of pregnant women whose first antenatal visit occurred before the fifth month of pregnancy. For the four states for which this was calculated, the percentages were between 58 and 85 per cent (Rice-Marquez *et al.* 1988).

From these programmes it is clear that, with supervision and some basic support, CHWs are able to provide a reasonable quality of service as measured by these outcomes. There seems no doubt that in relatively contained programmes guaranteeing supervision is both feasible and attained. However, national government programmes face enormous constraints of management, where weak infrastructures are bolstered by rules and regulations introduced to ensure uniformity and equity, but which actually result in rigidity, immobility and demoralization. In the large programmes where supervision is almost by definition sporadic, hampered by distances and lack of organization, there must be some doubt as to the service CHWs are able to provide. However, this should be seen within the context of the whole health service: CHWs are part of a system, and it is to that system we now turn.

References

Abbott, F. and MacMahon, R. (1985). *Teaching Health Care Workers: A Practical Guide*. Macmillan, London.

Aitkin, J. (1986). Point of view: to inject or not to inject. In Jayarao, K.S. and Patel, A.J. (eds), *Under the Lens*. Medico Friend Circle, New Delhi.

Bentley, C. (1989). Primary health care in northwestern Somalia: a case study *Social Science and Medicine*, 28, 10, 1019–30.

Berman, P., Gwatkin, D. and Burger, S. (1986). Community-based health workers: head start or false start towards health for all? PHN Technical Note 86-3, Washington: World Bank.

Bhattacharji, S. *et al.* (1986). Evaluating community health worker performance in India. *Health Policy and Planning*, 1, 3, 232–9.

Chandra, R. *et al.* (1980). Utilization of services of community health workers by the rural population. *Indian Journal of Medical Research*, 71, 6, 975–84.

Chowdhury, A.M.R. and Vaughan, J.P (1988). Perceptions of diarrhoea and the use of a homemade oral rehydration solution in rural Bangladesh. *Journal of Diarrhoeal Disease Research* 6, 1, 6–14.

Enge, K. *et al.* (1984). *Evaluation: Health Promoter Programs*, Ministry of Health, Lima. Management Sciences for Health, Boston USA.

Frankel, S. (1984). Peripheral health workers are central to PHC: lessons from PNG's aid posts. *Social Science and Medicine*, 19, 3, 279–90.

Gerein, N. (1988). Is growth monitoring worthwhile? *Health Policy and Planning*, 3, 3, 181–94.

Government of Somalia/Unicef (1986). *Review of Primary Health Care 1986*. Unicef/Ministry of Health, Somali Democratic Republic.

Gray, C. (1986). State-sponsored primary health care in Africa: the recurrent cost of performing miracles. *Social Science and Medicine*, 22, 3, 361–8.

Heggenhougen, K. *et al.* (1987) *Community Health Workers: the Tanzanian Experience*. Oxford University Press, Oxford.

Hongvivatana, T. *et al.* (1987). *A Study of Alternatives to the PHC Volunteer and Community Organization Strategy. A Final Report*. Mahidol University, Thailand.

Jacobson, H. *et al.* (1987). Time distribution of CHW activities: does curative care preclude preventive care? *Health Policy and Planning*, 2, 1, 85–9.

Kaseje, D. (1987). Characteristics and functions of CHWs in Saradidi, Kenya. *Annals of Tropical Medical Parasitology*, 81 (Supplement 1), 56–66.

Maru, R. (1983). The community health volunteer scheme in India – an evaluation. *Social Science and Medicine*, 17, 19, 1477–83.

Meche, H., Dibeya, T. and Bennett, J. (1984). The training and use of community health agents in Ethiopia. *Ethiopian Journal of Health Development*, 1, 1, 31–40.

O'Connor, R. *et al.* (1980). *Managing Health Systems in Developing Areas*. Lexington Books, Lexington, MA.

O'Dempsey, J. (1988). Health education and traditional cultures. Letter in *The Lancet* (II) 686.

Ofosu-Amaah, V. (1983). *National Experience in the Use of Community Health Workers: A Review of Current Issues and Problems*. Offset Publications, 71. WHO, Geneva.

Rice-Marquez, N, Baker, T. and Fischer, C. (1988). The community health worker: forty years of experience of an integrated primary rural health care system in Brazil. *The Journal of Rural Health*, 4, 1, 87–100.

Sales, A. (1977). Village health teams in Niger. Unpublished MSc dissertation, Diploma in Tropical Public Health, London School of Hygiene and Tropical Medicine.

Skeet, M. (1984). Community health workers: promoters or inhibitors of primary health care? *World Health Forum*, 5, 4, 291–5.

Sudsukh, V. (1982). *Inter-regional Study on Community Health Workers*. Ministry of Health, Thailand.

Taylor, D. (1986). *A Tale of Two Villages*. New Internationalist Publications, Oxford.

Werner, D. and Bower, B. (1982). *Helping Health Workers Learn*. The Hesperian Foundation, Palo Alto, CA.

WHO (1977). *The Primary Health Worker*. Experimental edition. WHO, Geneva.

Williams, G. (1986). A child survival revolution: prospects for Indonesia. *Prisma*, 40, 12–23.

4 | Links in a chain?

Although many national community health worker (CHW) programmes were planned almost like vertical programmes and grafted on to existing health infrastructures, they are nevertheless usually closely linked with health services. CHWs are also often expected to answer to – or consult with – a village health committee or other development institution within a community, linking with similar workers from other sectors, such as community development and agricultural extension workers. Finally, they are also expected to have close ties to traditional providers of care within their communities: indigenous practitioners of various kinds (herbalists, bone-setters, and so on) and also traditional midwives or birth attendants. To what extent are these links made? Who provides the role models for CHWs? Where do their loyalties lie? Let us look at each link in the chain: links with health services; with other sectors such as agriculture; with community organizations; and with traditional practitioners.

Links with health services

Reviewing the literature it becomes apparent that, with some notable exceptions (such as David Werner), it has been doctors such as Behrhorst, the Aroles, Chowdhury, and Antia who have instigated and implemented successful health schemes that have trained CHWs. And it is medical professionals who have persuaded policy-makers and politicians to support CHW programmes. The involvement of the nursing profession and other primary health care (PHC) workers in planning CHW schemes has been minimal, although it is nurses who most often train and supervise CHWs, sometimes aided by health inspectors and health assistants.

There is some evidence to suggest that CHW programmes were, in fact, often not initially welcomed by the nursing profession: 'Trained nursing staff became quite agitated when the community began to call the health aides the "new nurses" and began to demand more health services than the aides were trained or allowed to provide' (Marchione 1984). Certainly CHWs often identify with nurses and aspire to take on their roles (Cumper and Vaughan 1985). Perhaps it is because nurses were rarely involved in planning for CHW programmes that they have been slow to understand the full potential of CHWs in PHC, and have thus tended to use them just as extra pairs of hands in the clinics. In Botswana initial suspicion of the CHW programme gave way to acceptance as professional staff realized their potential as extra human resources in the clinics, and diverted the programme to suit their own ends.

This tendency to ignore the nurses is indicative of a much wider malaise. The medical profession has traditionally accorded only low status to the nursing profession; until the late 1980s nurses were relegated a back seat in the promotion of PHC, despite the fact that in many Third World countries it was they who were the majority of front-line workers providing PHC services.

Lack of consultation with nurses in PHC policy formulation and implementation has been exacerbated, however, by trends within the nursing profession itself, which has been seeking in the last two decades to professionalize, to increase the number of nurse graduates and to improve management capabilities. As international communication and professional exchange has increased, so many Third World countries have been drawn into importing models of nurse training which are not appropriate or relevant to local conditions (Masson 1978). Initial training establishes attitudes to reinforce professional ethos through special uniforms, epaulettes, badges and caps, as well as through hierarchical working relationships, job differentiation, status and aspirations, all of which run counter to ideas in PHC and the role of CHWs in the community. Professionals usually pursue their work in institutions, and pride in their work often translates into attitudes of superiority over staff with lower qualifications and less training. It is not surprising that many CHWs, who work closely with nurses and other primary health professionals, aspire to be like their nearest role models, and that they distance themselves from their communities. Working in clinics rather than making home visits legitimizes and increases their position as health workers.

Status admiration, however, does not obviate conflict. The potential for role strain in the PHC team is illustrated by Nichter's (1986) comparative analysis of two situations in India and Sri Lanka. Conflicts arose over skills, competence and status between doctors, different types of nurses and other health professionals. Medical officers tended to 'underplay the skills of field staff and jealously guard medical supplies'. Auxiliary nurse midwives felt threatened by CHWs, perhaps because of their own insecure knowledge base. In general, poorly trained and inadequately salaried nurses of low rank – who are often young and relatively inexperienced – may be the least able to work supportively with older, respected CHWs. Their discomfort is translated at worst into hostility, or a distortion of the CHWs' roles, making them nursing aides.

Health professionals' attitudes towards CHWs are also affected by their own training, which is usually based on biomedical, scientific principles that take little account of the cultural or material realities of people's lives. There are often enormous schisms in perception between CHWs and professional health staff, and because CHWs struggle to take on the standpoint of the professionals they may distance themselves even further from the communities in which they live, where beliefs and culture are likely to differ significantly from those of the educated health professionals.

Government health services employ health professionals to provide a service in both urban and rural areas. Most are taught in urban medical or nursing schools, and in spite of some attempts to make curricula more appropriate to national – rather than international – needs most training remains strongly biomedical and biased towards the treatment of illness. It is not surprising, then, that health professionals based in rural facilities see their most important function as providing a service (both preventive and curative) in a fixed facility which is open on a regular basis. If such a facility has a relatively regular supply of drugs it is likely to be used, although utilization rates may differ quite considerably. From some facilities, outreach visits may be made to more distant parts of the catchment area,

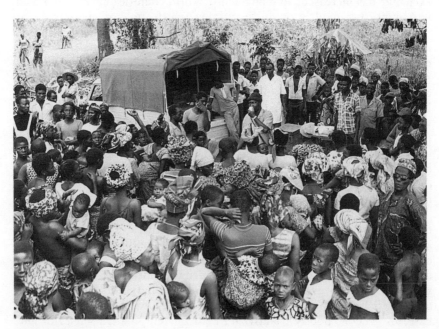

4   CHWs mobilize the population to gather for an outreach immunization visit from the health services. Photo: WHO by H. Anenden.

but this will depend on access to transport, and staff attitudes. Where outreach is not considered an essential part of routine services the importance of CHWs' roles within the communities will not be understood. The urgent need to retrain clinic-based nursing staff both in attitudes to community work and outreach is increasingly argued (Hammond 1987) but change occurs slowly. Even though nurse training courses have been adjusted to provide some teaching on PHC, the main emphasis remains on curative care, and the highest status is still accorded to nurses working in tertiary institutions. Under such circumstances the majority of nurses are ill equipped, in mind and function, to work positively in rural community services.

Not only are health professionals such as nurses often not technically prepared for working in peripheral health units, they may feel quite negative towards employment in primary care units. Simmonds (1989) argues that many governments have tended to neglect peripheral health workers, ignoring high levels of discontent. The personnel management problems that affect the routine working lives and prospects of health workers are legion, and the combination of government complacency and lack of resources for primary levels has deepened workers' dissatisfactions. It would be surprising if a demoralized workforce were able to offer its CHWs much support, much less a community-orientated example to emulate.

Given this, can CHWs bridge the gap between the primary health professionals and the community? Can they be the catalysts for community participation in health? Experience suggests not. A review of several health programmes in the Americas came to this conclusion:

The fact that most CHWs are paid and supervised by the health system, even though they may be selected from and by the community, tends to separate them from the community and identify them wholly with the formal system: they become the lowest-level staff rather than a link to the community (PAHO 1984).

Since more recent experience has shown that CHWs are, in fact, seldom selected by the community, it seems unlikely that they will be able to fulfil the PHC goal that they should be accountable to the community. Very few examples exist where communities control their own CHWs, either through funding or by overseeing their performance.

Yet even though CHWs tend to identify with the health service (and derive their status within the community because of this link) they need not necessarily be distanced from the community. Unlike other health professionals, CHWs come from the community in which they work, and, more importantly, they tend to remain there. One of the major weaknesses of many rural health infrastructures is the high turnover of personnel – with frequent transfers to other levels of the health service – resulting in a lack of continuity of care, and often limited professional interest and commitment to that community (Simmonds 1989). Besides providing a stable presence, CHWs may have added impact because of contacts with colleagues from other sectors, such as agricultural extension workers. And they may have ties with local voluntary organizations. Let us now look at these two links in the chain.

Links with other sectors

Other sectors – as well as the health sector – have introduced community-based workers to increase participation between government services and the community. Participatory policies focusing on the community have been tested in a variety of social programmes over the past forty years. During the 1980s, education, agriculture, housing, social work and community development programmes all struggled to achieve equitable distribution, reduce costs and develop basic services to meet people's needs (Macpherson 1982; Midgley *et al.* 1986). Community participation was a central theme of many of these programmes. In most cases, front-line workers were seen as the link between the professional staff and the community (Brekelbaum 1984), the mechanism through which community participation would take place (Paul 1987). The interpretation of what 'link' means in this context is, however, variable: for some it is a mechanism through which community demands are expressed and aspirations met; for others it is a mechanism through which support and information are both sought and given. The first derives from development goals, the second from service goals.

What is surprising is that, while there are many different kinds of community-based worker in different sectors, there is a dearth of comparative experience reported in the health literature. One rare paper compares extension workers from the three sectors in Botswana (Fortmann 1985), and Foster (1982) draws lessons for PHC from community development, regretting the fact that most PHC practitioners have not learned from the lessons of the community development movement. In exploring approaches to using front-line workers in community development and agriculture it is useful to keep in mind two themes: the ideological roots of the programmes; and the rationale for using community-based workers.

Community development workers

The community development approach was promoted and supported by heavy inputs of aid from the First World (the United States and Britain in particular) to Third World countries, after the Second World War. (Similar strategies were used by the French in Francophone countries under the *animation rurale* approach to grass roots development (Macdonald 1986).) For example, the British Colonial Office proposed community development as a way of helping the British African colonies prepare for independence by improving local government capabilities and developing their economies (Colonial Office 1958). A number of modest national community development programmes launched in Africa in the 1950s established village development committees, self-help projects, and literacy and vocational training programmes. The massive community development programme in India

> was intended to galvanize millions of villagers all over the country to articulate their 'felt' needs and to participate in programmes of social and economic development. The efforts and resources of the people and the state were to be combined for this purpose (Madan 1987).

Most community development programmes included development agents of some sort, part of whose role was to initiate or encourage community participation where it was not forthcoming, 'by the use of techniques for arousing and stimulating it' (Colonial Office 1958). Usually paid by government, these agents were trained as multi-purpose workers and sent to villages to assist in the development process at this level. Their skills were expected to be in communication, motivation and organization, with an ability to draw on technicians from specific sectors to help them implement projects. They were usually males, and their main function was to try to improve the lot of the downtrodden and less fortunate, and to 'modernize' the community (Holdcroft 1978).

Several observers have pointed to differing ideological rationales behind the financing of community development programmes in the Third World. Contrary to officially stated aims, it has been suggested that community development was a British attempt to 'maximise the extension and growth of colonial penetration and control' (Macpherson 1982). Holdcroft (1978) says that it was because of the perceived threat of revolution in South-east Asia after 'loss' of China to the Communists that the United States of America promoted the community development programme in India after independence. In Latin America, Ugalde (1985) argues that community development programmes were introduced to generate much-needed support from the rural masses for both the liberal democracies and the authoritarian regimes of the region.

By the early 1970s scepticism about the community development approach abounded. Three broad lessons have relevance for CHW programmes. First, participation proved to be an elusive goal and, if it occurred, rarely included the poorest segments of rural society. Village development workers, who were often secondary-school leavers, tended to identify with the traditional village elite to whom most of the benefits of development projects accrued. Hence they reinforced paternalistic and centralist traditions (Holdcroft 1978).

Second, national decision-makers were naive in believing that community development was an apolitical approach to rural development. Basic conflicts of class, land ownership and urban dominance were pervasive and directly influenced – and often diverted – the work of community workers (Manghezi 1976). Third, the move from local or 'pilot' projects to regional or national programmes was shown to be fraught with difficulties. Sussman

(1980) describes how a successful project in India, which specifically concentrated on organizational mechanisms in order to ensure replicability, was nevertheless diluted when it attempted to achieve high coverage. The very points that made the programme viable and successful (good supply and support systems, co-ordination between sectors, flexibility and responsiveness to local needs) were lost in the eagerness to extend the programme to a much larger population. Because the political pressures for expansion were great, operational quality was abandoned in favour of quantity and rapid expansion. Today the community development programme in India seeks to maximize the benefits of government activities rather than to promote community involvement (Madan 1987).

The extent to which CHWs have been involved with community development workers differs from country to country, but in general the contacts seem few and far between. Community development workers, in general, have higher educational levels, longer training courses and are paid as civil servants by governments. For all these reasons, Fortmann (1985) argues that they are less effective than CHWs: they are fewer in number and therefore have responsibility for larger populations; and they are transferable and therefore are less in contact with the community within which they work.

Yet community development workers and CHWs often have quite similar goals. It was partly because of this that the roles of community development worker and village health worker in Zimbabwe have been merged, and village health workers are being upgraded as community development workers under the Ministry of Women's Affairs and Community Development, instead of under the Ministry of Health. This programme was started in the late 1980s, and faces enormous constraints, but it is a rare example of a national programme trying to merge the roles of community-based workers.

Agricultural extension workers

The agricultural extension approach has also largely been a post-Second World War phenomenon. Early extension activities were mainly associated with export crops (for example, rubber, sugar, tea and coffee) with little attention to traditional food crops. After independence, many countries broadened the emphasis of agricultural extension to include peasant farmers, and promoted the agricultural extension worker (AEW) as a community-based worker who could advise and assist farmers in new methods leading to higher crop production, higher per capita incomes and increased foreign exchange reserves (Swanson 1984). However, traditional extension methods focused mainly on richer farmers, assuming that they were more able to take the risk inherent in innovation. The theory was that their increased wealth and example would 'trickle down' to the poorer members of the community (Garforth 1982).

One debate in the agricultural extension literature has particular relevance for CHWs: it emphasizes a specific type of training, and the mechanisms for supervision. Born out of criticisms of the traditional methods used for training and supervising agricultural extension workers, a system of training and visit (T & V) was devised in 1977 (Benor *et al.* 1984). T & V is based on four principles:

- Singleness of purpose. (AEWs have a purely advisory role. They do not write reports, supply seeds, fertilizers or credit.
- Concentration on key tasks. AEWs learn a couple of key tasks or messages every two weeks in a day of training, to ensure relevance of work and not to overburden them with more information than they can handle.
- Regular and predictable schedules. AEWs have a rigid schedule of visits to contact farmers and for training and supervision, usually based on a two-week rotation.
- Face-to-face communication and feedback. AEWs are the link between the farmers and the agricultural sector.

There has been much debate about the benefits of T & V (Howell 1982; 1983), one of several criticisms being that it is very expensive (Moore 1984) since experience shows that T & V is only successful when all the above mutually reinforcing elements are simultaneously implemented (Heaver 1984). There may well be lessons here for CHW schemes. One attempt to look at the implications of T & V for population, health and nutrition workers concluded that, although there are inherent differences between health and agriculture, some aspects of T & V could usefully be adapted (Heaver 1984).

Heaver compares four programmes – in India, the Philippines (one governmental and one non-governmental) and Indonesia – which use CHWs (both paid and volunteers). He scores each programme for managerial effectiveness, and from an analysis of performance and resource-uses in each programme he illustrates a basic paradox of volunteer systems: that they are often adopted for cheapness, yet without close support and supervision – which can be prohibitively expensive – they are ineffective. A tightly managed outreach system which employs smaller numbers of paid workers may be more expensive but more cost-effective.

Selective targeting of households, task concentration, and more in-service training are all lessons from T & V that could benefit CHW schemes, and there may be others. However, T & V is a very hierarchical method of organizing the delivery of information and technical inputs to scattered rural recipients, and this is not how most CHW programmes are conceived. Even national CHW programmes envisage a participatory role for community members rather than making them mere recipients of services and information.

Agricultural extension remains an important policy in most countries, and debates about improving programmes cover issues familiar to those concerned with health worker programmes. There are lessons to be learned from technical analyses such as Heaver's (1984), and also from debates about, for example, motivation: not only what motivates AEWs, with concomitant issues of recruitment, training, selection, supervision and career structure (Fortmann 1985), but also what motivates farmers to adopt innovations (Garforth 1982) and whether richer farmers continue to be favoured by the T & V system (Feder *et al.* 1984).

Similar questions can be asked of CHWs' motivations: which of their health education messages are likely to be adopted, and which community members they are most likely to contact. Fortmann's (1985) comparison of agricultural demonstrators, assistant community development officers and family welfare educators in Botswana concluded that the other two sectors could learn from the experience in health. She found that the family welfare educators who were selected from their own communities were more acceptable to these communities and were working better than the other cadres which were imposed externally, and for whom the decisions 'to hire, fire, transfer, promote or send for training are all made at the centre' (Fortmann 1985). Of course, it could also be argued that family welfare educators were more acceptable because of the nature of the services which they offered.

In summary, although the rationale for their front-line workers had different origins in the health, community development and agriculture sectors, there are strikingly familiar themes in all three. The pursuit of participation and community involvement is common to all and remains elusive to all; the political environment is, on the whole, ignored or neglected, yet influences everything from distribution to who contacts whom; and the dilemma of replication – expanding from small to national coverage – remains a mutual predicament.

Links with community organizations

A number of studies have noted that CHWs often have a history of active involvement in local voluntary organizations, so although CHWs identify with the health professionals, they still have ties with community-level voluntary organizations. In Botswana, family welfare educators are members of voluntary organizations, and in both Sri Lanka (Perera *et al.* 1988) and Peru (Enge *et al.* 1984) CHWs play a part in a number of different local organizations outside the health field. In Thailand it was noted that CHWs who are members of community organizations performed their health activities more effectively (Sudsukh *et al.* 1982).

What are examples of these local organizations? The local government structures, such as the district councils in Botswana, form part of the state's administrative system. Other local institutions exist, too, and most countries have a number of modern institutions at local level which have ties to similar institutions at higher levels. These include trade unions, farmers'

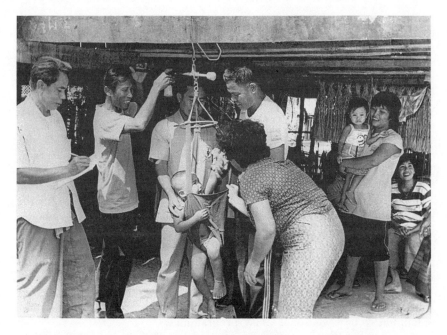

5 Village communicators and volunteers help health service staff weigh babies in Thailand. Photo: WHO/Ministry of Public Health, Thailand.

associations and village development committees, as well as the lowest tiers of mass organizations – such as Cuba's Committees for the Defence of the Revolution or Tanzanian villages' ten cells (households). There are also often traditional institutions such as the *kgotla* of Botswana, and a variety of religious organizations, all of which may exert considerable authority in a local area, although in many parts of the less-developed world their power has waned as governments have increased their control over and regulation of people's lives.

Other organizations may include, for example, mothers' clubs, burial societies, parent and teacher associations and women's secret societies which may embody both traditional and modern norms. Such groups thrive where their members see some benefit to themselves or their environment. In Botswana and Zimbabwe, for example, studies show that burial societies have been enormously successful, largely because they meet a perceived need (financial assistance at the time of a death in the family), have no competing organizations, and are able to apply individual sanctions against members who break their rules (Brown *et al.* 1982).

These are examples of voluntary organizations which have been initiated within the community and whose leaders are often women. They contrast sharply with the largely ineffective health committees that have been set up in many countries, supposedly to support CHWs, and which have largely been imposed on communities from the outside – with scant attention either to the mechanisms of participation and support, or their social and political composition.

Members of village (or urban) health committees often have only the vaguest idea of the purpose of such committees, and certainly do not perceive them as meeting an agreed need. In Mexico one observer said the village health committee members 'hardly know the responsibility invested in them and even less the role they have to play' (Navarro 1987). They seldom have control of resources, and where money is involved, abuse and mismanagement of funds may occur, as has happened in some villages in The Gambia, for example (Cham *et al.* 1987). In another programme in Senegal, where the treasurer on the health committee was initially the only member to have control over the finances, his susceptibility to requests for loans from his relatives clearly threatened to undermine the programme's viability. This was eventually overcome by training all village health committee members in the operation of the health facilities and their financial management. This meant that they were in a good position to support their CHWs and, in this instance, traditional midwives (Doan *et al.* 1984). This latter example, however, is from a programme which received large inputs of technical and financial aid from external donors, a situation unfamiliar to most national CHW programmes.

Members of village health committees often lack leadership skills as they seldom receive any training in community development or participation. Furthermore, membership of such committees is often highly biased – a fact that tends to be overlooked by the health system. In many villages, class, caste, gender and age are important criteria for choice of membership. Committees made up of women are likely to be of low status in the village hierarchy, even though they may be more active in targeting PHC activities towards women and children. Where men and women sit on a committee, the men are likely to represent the traditional political power of the community, and to dominate any proceedings.

Unfortunately, members of village health committees may be seen by the local health staff simply as an adjunct to the health system, and may be used by staff (or CHWs) to help implement minor health activities without necessarily being given adequate credit for their assistance. In one urban area of Jamaica, health committee members helped to raise and allocate funds for improving the health centre, but their meetings were dominated by the professional staff who viewed them merely as 'assistants' (PAHO 1984).

It is important to ask who makes up the community. A village community is a matrix, composed of many different strata and different political factions, with historical differences between groups. There are also often multi-religious or ethnic groups. Villages in Sri Lanka may contain both Muslims and Buddhists, and health volunteers of one group will not, on the whole, be able to visit homes of the other group. Social and economic relationships are overlain by a set of local institutions, both formal and informal, traditional and modern. All too often attempts to set up new institutions such as health committees have not taken into account the heterogeneity of social groups or the existence of local organizations, and therefore have not been successful. A review of village health committees in Botswana showed that very few of these committees are active, and that 90 per cent of the village population did not know why they selected members for such committees (Owuor-Omondi *et al.* 1987).

In one village in Botswana the health committee was paralysed because of its conflict with the village development committee. The tension stemmed from the belief of members of the village development committee (who were mainly members of the opposition political party) that any campaign or activity within the village implied support for the government (Owuor-Omondi *et al.* 1987). In Colombia a complex and aggressive political system means that loyalties to particular interests may be hard won (and lost). In Sri Lanka local institutions are highly political, and villagers often have to seek patronage before they can apply for jobs or for places on courses.

At the end of the day, however, it is fairly clear from the health literature that participation in health programmes tends to be narrowly interpreted with only two objectives in mind: either to get communities involved in donating time, labour or material for particular ends; or else to get communities to utilize the services that have largely been designed and delivered by the health system. Professionals seek participation as a means of enhancing the utilization of health services, not as a way of challenging their own control over planning and delivery. They therefore emphasize institutional care more than outreach and continue to control, rather than have a partnership with, paraprofessionals or non-professionals. All this is a long way from the original ideas of participation, where people were to have a right to participate in decisions about their health. Clearly it affects CHWs' involvement with communities: mobilization for health campaigns, regular immunization, and follow-up of non-compliers may be all that professionals expect from CHWs. It would be unusual, then, if CHWs were able to play a more radical role within their own community with regard to initiating participation.

Links with traditional practitioners

If CHWs in national programmes identify closely with the health professionals at their side, how close are their ties likely to be with traditional practitioners or midwives in the community? Some, in fact, may have been traditional practitioners, although in national programmes this is not usually the case.

For all the rhetoric since the Alma Ata declaration of 1978, links between government health services and the traditional sector remain extremely tenuous. Even with traditional midwives, who in many less-developed countries are still the main source of help in childbirth, links have been limited to short training programmes. Although CHWs are often trained in delivery skills the extent to which they actually assist in labour is limited (although this differs markedly from country to country). In Sri Lanka, for example, even the public health midwife seldom attends births because most women deliver in institutions.

The shift towards PHC gave credence to ideas about the benefits of home deliveries by traditional birth attendants (TBAs) or traditional midwives, and many countries, with assistance from WHO and Unicef, have introduced short training courses for women who are recognized in their communities as the main source of help in labour. Such courses typically last only one to three weeks; students learn family planning methods, antiseptic techniques and detection of high-risk pregnancies. They are often rewarded at the end with a simple maternity kit.

There is, however, increasing scepticism about the usefulness of such courses. Jeffery *et al.* (1988), writing about northern India, observe that *dai* training programmes have failed to comprehend *dais* and birthing practices in the wider framework of childbearing. There are enormous structural constraints on women, who are valued essentially for their childbearing capacity but who do not control any of the decisions that affect pregnancy, such as the use of antenatal services, acceptance of tetanus toxoid, or the need for rest and adequate nutrition. Local understanding about childbearing – which includes strong notions of shame and pollution – are also not taken into account. Even if *dais* have been trained by health professionals, and retain and use their new knowledge (which is extremely difficult to ascertain) they may be limited in where they can help:

> The Harijan dai is welcome only while the new mother is herself unclean; the Caste Hindu dai is tainted by her work. Only for a Muslim among Muslims or a Harijan among Harijans, and then not always, are the barriers between a dai and her client at a minimum. Government health staff, as urban superiors, are socially distant in one direction, while the dai, as a polluted menial, is socially distant in the other.

One analysis of methods used for training traditional midwives in Mexico is devastating in its criticism (Jordan 1989). Drawing on experience from years of ethnographic fieldwork with Maya midwives in Yucatan, and on participation in government-sponsored training courses for indigenous midwives, Jordan suggests that such courses have failed miserably to meet their objectives. In her analysis of instructional methods she draws attention to inappropriate modes of teaching that put emphasis on definitions – which are empty rhetoric – and irrelevant messages. This last is illustrated vividly:

> In Yucatan, as in many parts of the world, women believe that the most fertile time is immediately before and after menstruation, because at that time 'the uterus is open'. Women who want to avoid pregnancy

will have intercourse at midcycle when they believe the uterus to be closed – exactly at the most fertile time. The medical staff, however, were not aware of this belief, and anyway, there was no space for discussing it in the lesson plan. So the family planning course failed to impart the single piece of information which could be expected to have significant impact on contraceptive behaviour.

Jordan does not gloss over the difficulties of imparting knowledge which challenges traditional views but argues that, at the end of the course, midwives will graduate successfully because they have learned to give their trainers the 'right' answers, although these will bear little resemblance to how they will later practise. She contrasts this didactic mode of learning (good for learning *how to talk about doing something*) with the apprenticeship mode of learning (good for learning *how to do something*).

Moreover, even where training is apparently appropriate, the links between the traditional midwives and the health services may be more with professional staff than with CHWs. A programme in Zimbabwe was described as successful because of the positive relationship between maternity assistants at health clinics and the *vanambuya*, who were trained once a fortnight over a five- or six-month period:

> The great advantage of the programme is that it is locally administered. The maternity assistants get to know the TBAs well, and in many of the clinics collaboration between them has been enthusiastic. Maternity assistants noted that many TBAs have been encouraging women to go to antenatal clinics, and to take children for immunizations. Maternity assistants, who train the TBAs, have a detailed knowledge of local conditions. This is important because beliefs and practices differ quite markedly from one part of the province to another (Booker, quoted in WHO 1984).

The relevance of the above information for CHWs comes in the explanation of how it stems from differing world views, which are described as clashing views of social relationships and of bodily structures and processes. Health professionals see themselves as upholders of modern, scientific thought, representing official views. As we have already seen, CHWs take these professionals as their role models and are therefore likely to distance themselves from traditional customs with which they may still be in contact, or to experience considerable conflict in their relationships with traditional midwives, or even ordinary community members. In Sri Lanka, health volunteers' complaints about the communities' reliance on traditional remedies (which they also admit to using), and the dismissive attitude of the professional staff to such remedies, probably reflects this sense of conflict. It is certainly generally claimed that health professionals are often pejorative about traditional beliefs and remedies. Where such negative attitudes exist, community members may see them as indicating a lack of respect, which clearly does little to foster co-operation or participation.

The CHW is part of an environment influenced by the existence of many institutions and systems: the health sector is only part of the whole. However, it is the health sector which ultimately defines the parameters within which the CHW lives and works. Although CHWs come from communities and tend to remain there, they seldom establish strong links either with other extension agents working in that community, or with community organizations, or with traditional health practitioners. The influence of health professionals' understanding of health, attitudes towards communities and perception of the CHW's role has been so pervasive that CHWs are now securely fastened to the apron strings of the formal health system. In the next chapter we look more closely at the one aspect of CHW programmes in which the health system has sought directly to involve communities: their financing.

References

Benor, D. *et al.* (1984). *Agricultural Extension: The Training and Visit System.* World Bank, Washington, DC.

Brekelbaum, T. (1984) The use of paraprofessionals in rural development. *Community Development Journal*, 19, 4, 232–45.

Brown, C. *et al.* (1982). *A Study of Local Institutions in Kgatleng District, Botswana.* Applied Research Unit, Ministry of Local Government and Lands, Gaborone.

Cham, K. *et al.* (1987). Social organization and political factionalism: PHC in The Gambia. *Health Policy and Planning*, 2, 3, 214–26.

Colonial Ofice (1958). *Community Development: A Handbook.* HMSO, London.

Cumper, G. and Vaughan, J. (1985). Community health aides at the crossroads. *World Health Forum*, 6, 4, 365–7.

Doan, R.L. *et al.* (1984). *Local Institutional Development for Primary Health Care.* Rural Development Committee, Cornell University, New York, USA.

Enge, K. *et al.* (1984). *Evaluation: Health Promoter Programs.* Ministry of Health, Lima. Management Sciences for Health, Boston, USA.

Feder, G. *et al.* (1984). *The Training and Visit System: An Analysis of Operations and Effects.* Discussion paper 14, Agricultural Administration Unit, Overseas Development Institute, London.

Fortmann, L. (1985). Factors affecting agricultural and other rural extension services in Botswana. *Agricultural Administration*, 18, 1, 13–23.

Foster, G. (1982). Community development and primary health care: their conceptual similarities. *Medical Anthropology*, 6, 3, 183–95.

Garforth, C. (1982). Reaching the rural poor: a review of extension strategies and methods. In Jones, G.E. and Rolls, M.J. (eds), *Progress in Rural and Community Development*, Vol 1. John Wiley and Sons, London.

Hammond, M. (1987). Clinic-based health care auxiliaries: an overlooked but essential category? *Health Policy and Planning*, 2, 3, 234–41.

Heaver, R. (1984). *Adapting the Training and Visit System for Family Planning, Health and Nutrition Programmes.* Staff working paper no. 662. World Bank, Washington, DC.

Holdcroft, L. (1978). *The Rise and Fall of Community Development in Developing Countries, 1950–65: A Critical Analysis and Annotated Bibliography.* Rural Development Paper no. 2, Michigan State University, Ann Arbor.

Howell, J. (1982). *Managing Agricultural Extension: The T and V System in Practice.* Discussion paper no. 8, Agricultural Administration Unit, Overseas Development Institute, London.

Howell, J. (1983). *Strategy and Practice in the T and V System of Agricultural Extension.* Discussion paper no. 10, Agricultural Administration Unit, Overseas Development Institute, London.

Jeffery, P. *et al.* (1988). *Labour Pains and Labour Power.* Zed Press, London.

Jordan, B. (1989). Cosmopolitical obstetrics: some insights from the training of traditional midwives. *Social Science and Medicine,* 28, 9, 925–37.

Macdonald, J. (1986). Participatory evaluation and planning as an essential part of community development. PhD thesis, Dept of Education, University of Manchester, UK.

Macpherson, S. (1982). *Social Policy in the Third World.* Wheatsheaf Books, Hassocks, Sussex.

Madan, T.N. (1987). Community involvement in health policy: socio-structural and dynamic aspects of health beliefs. *Social Science and Medicine,* 25, 6, 615–20.

Manghezi, A. (1976). *Class, Elite and Community in African Development.* The Scandinavian Institute for African Studies, Uppsala, Sweden.

Marchione, T. (1984). Evaluating primary health care and nutrition programmes in the context of national development. *Socials Science and Medicine,* 19, 3, 225–35.

Masson, V. (1978). Nursing for export – let the buyer beware. *International Nursing Review,* 25, 4.

Midgley, J. *et al.* (1986). *Community Participation, Social Development and the State.* Methuen, London.

Moore, M. (1984). Institutional development, the World Bank, and India's new agricultural extension programme. *Journal of Development Studies,* 20, 4, 303–17.

Navarro, F. (1987). Primary health care in social solidarity services of the Mexican Institute of Social Security. Paper presented at a conference sponsored by the Rockefeller Foundation at Bellagio, Italy, 26–30 October.

Nichter, M. (1986). The primary health center as a social system: PHC, social status, and the issue of team-work in South Asia. *Social Science and Medicine.* 23, 4, 347–55.

Owuor-Omondi, L. *et al.* (1987). *Village Health Committees: Viable Instruments of Community Mobilisation for Primary Health Care?* National Health Status Evaluation Monograph Series, 4. Ministry of Health, Gaborone.

PAHO (1984). *Community Participation in Health and Development in the Americas: An Analysis of Selected Case Studies.* Scientific Publication, 473. PAHO, Washington, DC.

Paul, S. (1987). *Community Participation in Development Projects.* Discussion Paper no. 6. World Bank, Washington, DC.

Perera, M. *et al.* (1988). *Health Volunteers in Sri Lanka: Why Do They Volunteer?* Marga Institute, Colombo, and Evaluation and Planning Centre, London School of Hygiene and Tropical Medicine.

Simmonds, S. (1989). Human resource development: the management, planning and training of health personnel. *Health Policy and Planning,* 4, 3, 187–96.

Sudsukh, V. *et al.* (1982). *Inter-regional Study on Community Health Workers.* Ministry of Health, Bangkok.

Sussman, G. (1980). The pilot project and the choice of an implementing strategy: community development in India. In Grindle, M. (ed), *Politics and Policy Implementation in the Third World.* Princeton University Press, Princeton, NJ.

Swanson, B. (1984). *Agricultural Extension. A reference manual.* Food and Agriculture Organization, Rome.

Ugalde, A. (1985). Ideological dimensions of community participation in Latin American health programs. *Social Science and Medicine*, 21, 1, 41–53.

WHO (1984). The supervision of traditional birth attendants (TBAs). Unpublished paper HMD/NUR/84.1, Division of Health Manpower Development, WHO, Geneva.

5 | Sustaining community health worker programmes: who pays?

There is no doubt that many policy-makers in ministries of health assumed that community health workers (CHWs) would be an inexpensive way of extending health services, and on the surface this seemed plausible. If they were paid at all, their salaries were low, their training was short, and in many countries most of the initial training costs were met by outside agencies such as Unicef. If they had to be supplied with medicines, such supplies were usually minimal.

When planning CHW programmes little account was taken of their likely recurrent costs and their financing implications. It was assumed that communities would somehow pay for the services of CHWs, or that their costs would be absorbed into health budgets, and there was little discussion of the real costs of such programmes. Nor was much consideration given to the fact that CHWs trained for short periods were only effective if they were supported; and very few Ministries of Health calculated the costs (or even the feasibility) of supervision before they implanted CHW programmes.

The failure to sustain these programmes adequately has only become apparent as a result of experience with them, and as the health sector's resource constraints have bitten into the provision of all services – especially those at the periphery. These problems have generated a new concern with guaranteeing the continuity of CHW programmes: 'sustainability'. This concept has two aspects: how to improve the use of available resources by achieving greater cost-effectiveness in health activities; and how to secure new ways of financing health activities. It is perhaps too easy to focus on the lack of financial resources and to ignore the importance of other ways of improving sustainability. A programme in Nigeria, for example, reduced CHW attrition by improving career opportunities and providing more supportive supervision – demonstrating that 'money isn't always the key ingredient for improved sustainability' (Stinson 1987).

Let us start to consider the issue by exploring the costs of CHW programmes.

Community health worker programme costs

Costs fall into several different categories: the investment costs of training, and perhaps provision of facilities; and the recurrent costs of CHWs' salaries, supplies and supervision. They vary according to the type of programme, and different categories of costs may be borne by different groups: donor, health services, or community.

Basic training is generally provided at district or regional level by nurses or other primary health care (PHC) workers who are often expected to teach CHWs as part of their routine work. This is particularly true when training of CHWs occurs in a local health facility. Local training cuts down the costs of transport, food and accommodation. The differences can be quite marked, as shown by Table 3, which compares the cost of sending a village health worker out of the district to regional-level training with training done at a local health centre. Clearly, locally conducted short blocks (one-week courses over a period of time) appear to be 80 per cent less expensive than training at the regional level over a period of four months (de Savigny *et al.* 1988). It is unfortunately rare for national CHW programmes to devolve training to local levels, however, and therefore the costs are probably higher than is necessary. The fact that donors have often supported these training costs has hampered analysis of cost factors.

Table 3 Costs of training a village health worker, Tanzania (shillings).

	Regional level	Local level
Transport	2,000	438
Food and allowances	18,600	2,500
Salaries	984	1,438
Materials	428	294
Total	22,012	4,670

Source: de Savigny *et al.* (1988)

The cost of training also depends on the length of the course, the number of teachers and the number of trainees. A hypothetical costing based on experience in Swaziland explored the likely cost per CHW of a 'low-cost CHW' trained for three months and expected to work part-time, and a 'high-cost CHW' trained for six months and expected to work full-time. The two types of CHW were assumed to have different skills (for example, the high-cost CHW was allowed to prescribe from a limited range of drugs, whereas the low-cost CHW had no drugs), to receive different salaries, and to receive different degrees of supervision and in-service training (that is, more for the high-cost CHW). It was assumed that a group of thirty low-cost and twenty high-cost CHWs were trained at the same time by two and three teachers, respectively. Basic training cost were estimated to be 450 emalangeni (E) (US $220) per low-cost CHW and E1080 (US $520) per high-cost CHW in 1984–5 prices – equivalent to 35 per cent of the total cost of each less-skilled CHW and 31 per cent of the total cost of each higher-skilled CHW (Gilson 1987). Given this relative expense of basic training it is essential to ensure not only that the CHWs are trained in appropriate skills but also that the training is successful in preparing them to work effectively within communities. Ineffective training is a waste of time, effort and money.

Perhaps of most importance to the overall sustainability of CHW programmes is the cost of support and supervision. The costs of supervision are seldom considered for any level of the health service, let alone for CHWs. In his comparison of health projects with the agricultural training and visit (T & V) system, Heaver (1984) suggests that the experience from T & V shows that, once supervision ratios fall below one supervisor per eight CHWs, effectiveness also falls sharply. However, where supervisory ratios actually reach these levels, or higher, the costs are often prohibitive. The lessons for large-scale volunteer systems are clear: while they appear cheap to initiate, effective supervision is extremely expensive.

Two hypothetical costings, from Zambia (Harnmeijer 1988) and from Swaziland (Gilson 1987) explore the cost of supervision and in-service training within CHW programmes.

Supervision costs

In Zambia, CHWs are assumed to receive twelve supervision days per year (one visit per month) from the staff of the local rural health centre, plus one annual visit from a district staff member. They also receive a one-week refresher course at the rural health centre every year. (From Harnmeijer's (1989) study of forty Zambian CHWs we know that in reality supervision levels are much lower – more like one-and-a-half visits per annum!) In Swaziland, the frequency of supervision and in-service training is assumed to differ according to the type of CHW. Low-cost CHWs receive one supervisory visit per month from a nurse from the local health facility and attend two in-service training courses per year (of one day each), where they are taught by a nursing sister; higher-cost CHWs get two supervision visits per month from the local health facility and attend four in-service training courses per year (of one day each), where they are taught by a doctor. This pattern of support is assumed to be 'best practice', that is, the ideal, and not the reality. The composition of the cost per CHW in all three cases is shown in Tables 4 and 5.

The relative expense of frequent supervision is shown by the fact that, in each case, its cost represents over one-quarter of the total cost for each CHW: 29 per cent of the Swazi high-cost CHW, 37 per cent of the Swazi low-cost CHW, and 40 per cent of Zambian CHW. Whether money is well spent on frequent supervision depends on the quality of the contact made; in Colombia, although CHWs receive frequent supervision, the quality is

Table 4 Hypothetical annual recurrent costs per community health worker, Zambia (1986 kwacha).

		Formal system	Community	
1	CHW allowance		240	
2.1	Drugs	1120		1 CHW kit = K560, 2 kits per year for 250 pop.
2.2	Med. equip.	25		
2.3	Stationery	75		
2.4	Misc. equipment	25		
3	Bicycle spares/deprec.	300		
4.1	Shelter, maintenance	0	15	
4.2	Pit latrine	0	5	
4.3	Furniture	0	0	
5	Training refresher course			5 days at rural health centre with district
	Food, material K15/day/cap	75		facilitator
				Facilitator transport, 8 × 180 km 1440
				salary, 6 × 30 180
				subsistence, 5 × 60 300
				Driver salary, 6 × 10 60
				subsistence, 5 × 40 200
				1 RHC staff salary, 5 × 15 75
	If 4 CHWs trained: 2255/4	564		Total 2255
6	Supervision by RHC			
6.1	Salary	180		K.15/day
				12 visits/year
6.2	Subsistence	0		
	for 1 RHC staff			
6.3	Motorcycle 12 × 50 km	960		K1.6/km, spares, fuel, maintenance, depreciation
7	Supervision by district	562		1 × year
	Supervising group of 4 CHWs			
8	Referral		80	oxen hire for transport patient
	Subtotals	3886	340	
	Total:	4226		

Source: Harnmeijer (1988)

poor, and so the resources used in supervision are not utilized in a cost-effective way.

In-service training costs

In the hypothetical examples of Zambia and Swaziland, the cost of in-service training as a proportion of total cost per CHW varies substantially. In Zambia, 15 per cent of total cost is spent on in-service training, but in both cases in Swaziland under 2 per cent is spent. The difference partly reflects varying practices – the Zambian CHWs are assumed to receive a

Table 5 Hypothetical costing of community health workers based on Swaziland data and 'best practice' principles (1984–5 emalangeni)[1].

	Low-cost CHW[2]	High-cost CHW[3]
Salary	240	750
Drugs	0	500
Other recurrent	100	0
Supervision	480	950
In-service training	25	55
Basic training	450	1,080
Total	E1,295	E3,335

[1] The Swaziland data used are known costs of salaries, transport, etc., known practice with respect to length of training (low-cost CHW) and distance travelled; 'best practice' is assumed with respect to high-cost CHWs (who do not exist in Swaziland), and frequency of supervision and in-service training.
[2] Low-cost CHWs are expected to work only part-time, have preventive/educative functions and work from their homes.
[3] High-cost CHWs are expected to work full-time and in addition to preventive/promotive functions carry a limited range of drugs. They also work from their homes.

Source: Gilson (1987)

period of five days' training in a health facility, whilst the Swazi CHWs are assumed to receive only two or four days' training in a group of thirty (low-cost) CHWs or twenty (high-cost) CHWs – and each only a day at a time. Cost differences probably also reflect the varying cost of transport, the number of trainers and the trainers' salaries in the two countries. Which system is better is not clear, as both the cost and the effectiveness of training must be judged. If, as in Colombia, trainers in Zambia are themselves badly trained and uninterested, then the cost of the training may not be justified. On the other hand, if CHWs are better equipped and better motivated to perform their tasks in the community as a result of the training, then spending more on in-service training than is done at present in Swaziland, for example, could be seen to be a justifiable investment. As noted earlier, assessing sustainability does not simply involve considering the costs of the CHW programme but also depends on whether the expenditures are justified by the resulting benefits.

Cost considerations for planning community health worker programmes

In planning CHW programmes it is essential not only to estimate the total cost per CHW but also to consider the likely total cost of the programme as a whole. Although the cost per CHW may be substantially less than the cost of each rural health facility, for example, the total cost of the programme may still be beyond available resources (Berman *et al.* 1987). A lot depends on the number of CHWs trained. The problem of 'going to scale' from small project to nation-wide programme has been much discussed. From the data of the Niger primary health care (PHC) programme, Over (1986) suggests a possible two- or threefold increase of total recurrent costs in expanding the programme from the urban to the more remote areas. The increase mainly results from a higher attrition of village health teams (VHTs) and village health workers (VHWs) (due to lower valuation of their services, less support, and so on) and the consequent need to replace them, plus the higher average costs (per VHT) of expanding PHC services outside urban areas (as a result of higher input costs). Such scale effects include the increased supervision requirements. Although existing staff may be able to supervise some additional facilities and/or CHWs, in a national programme supervision requirements will probably increase so much that additional supervision staff will be necessary. Increased supervision needs will also have knock-on effects in terms of additional vehicle needs and other logistic support (Harnmeijer 1988).

Failure to consider the overall costs of CHW programmes undermines their implementation. In Jamaica, the number of CHWs was reduced by 62 per cent in the 1980s through redundancies and freezing training opportunities (Ennever et al. 1988). However, in calculating total resource requirements it is not appropriate simply to work out the cost per CHW and multiply by the number of CHWs to be trained. It is also necessary to consider the additional costs of introducing or expanding a CHW programme – by assessing the scale effects noted above. Too often it has been assumed that the only costs to consider are the salaries or the drugs, and that all other costs (including supervision) will somehow be absorbed. The consequence of this approach, especially when combined with cuts in real expenditure on health care, has been a failure to provide adequate supervision and support. When planning national programmes it is crucial to calculate the real cost of supervision, together with the cost of salaries, drugs, and so on, for each new CHW (that is, the CHWs' marginal cost to the health services), and this cost must be funded to ensure their effective employment. These marginal costs can also be used to help judge whether to invest resources in introducing or expanding CHW programmes, whether to put money into some alternative health programme – by comparing the relative costs and benefits of each.

Costs per contact

Another way of exploring the costs of any health activity is to consider the cost per contact, or cost per household (that is, average costs). In Botswana there are great differences in the average costs of health facilities, depending on how many (and which) cadres staff them, and the number of patients who visit them. Consultations with CHWs also vary enormously: in the Tombali area in Guinea-Bissau, consultations with village health workers or traditional midwives in village health units were 3.4 per capita in 1984, which differed from a national average of 0.7 for all health centres and hospitals (Chabot and Waddington 1987). In a non-governmental organization programme in Tanzania, annual attendances per capita were 9

– which is extremely high (the average per capita attendance at a general practitioner in the UK is 3.5 per year). Because there were so many visits (for free consultations), average costs per household were relatively low (103 Tanzanian shillings – 0.7 US $). Less than half of the development levy expected from all adult residents in the area would have been sufficient to meet the recurrent costs of the village health posts (de Savigny et al. 1988).

In the review of national programmes by Berman et al. (1987), the authors concluded that the average cost per service contact for CHWs in Indonesia, Thailand and China was well below the average cost for similar services at the next highest level in the delivery system. However, in Colombia the cost to the health service of a home visit by a CHW was the equivalent of US $1.80, twice the cost of an outpatient contact with a doctor in a health facility (de Salazar et al. 1987). Clearly, since CHWs only do an average of about four home visits per day, home visiting – even by low-paid CHWs – is relatively expensive for the health service. This assessment, however, ignores the cost advantages of CHWs to the community. The full cost of any programme is both the cost of providing a service plus the cost of using it. As CHWs are usually more accessible to communities than are the health facilities, the household cost of using the CHW service (for example, the time taken to 'reach' care) is probably much less than the cost of using more distant health units. If the Colombia study had included such household costs, the cost of a home visit, relative to that of an outpatient contact, would probably have been quite substantially reduced.

Of course, such comparisons have to be complemented by consideration of the relative effectiveness of the two types of contact. The home visit may be more effective in that the families visited are those most at risk yet those least likely to go to a health facility. But CHW services may not be comparable with those at higher levels of the health system (where a different range of services is provided), and the quality of the care that CHWs can provide is likely to be highly dependent on regular supervision. In areas where the primary level health facility is underutilized, because of poor supplies, staff attitudes, and so on, the chances of CHWs providing a more cost-effective service than the higher levels of the system are very remote. Concern for 'sustainability', therefore, requires planners to consider ways of enhancing cost-effectiveness, to ensure that value for money is obtained from the resources invested in CHW programmes.

Let us now look a little more closely at what has been learned about the financing of CHW programmes, and the possibilities for shifting some of this burden on to the communities themselves.

Who pays for community health worker programmes?

The training costs of CHW programmes are often met by donors such as Unicef. Donors may, for example, pay for materials (such as manuals), or may provide a daily allowance for the CHWs in training. But they rarely take responsibility for long-term · support for recurrent costs. Most governments provide and pay for the CHW trainers and, theoretically, cover the costs of supervision and support. Other costs are borne, in varying proportions, by the government and the communities: for example, the government may pay CHW salaries and provide medical supplies, while the community may build the health post from which the CHWs will work. Alternatively, the government may only be responsible for support and supervision, while the community will bear the cost of CHW remuneration and supplies (as happens in Senegal). In other instances CHWs may work voluntarily, the costs borne by themselves and their families.

Whatever the arrangements, there are often problems in maintaining financial support for CHW programmes. Where ministries are paying salaries, as in Botswana, Jamaica and Colombia, fewer CHWs are being trained than was originally envisaged. Maintaining supplies, supervision and other support is also difficult.

Government support for community health worker programmes

At one level, ministries of health face problems beyond their capacity to control. What was seen at the time of the Alma Ata declaration as being affordable has, in practice, been beyond the finances of many countries. A combination of lower economic growth and population increases led to falls in income and consumption per capita in many developing countries in the 1970s, followed by an even sharper drop in 1982. The proportion of public expenditure devoted to health in all less-developed countries halved from 6.1 per cent in 1972 to 3 per cent in 1982 – in contrast with the increase of 2 per cent (to 11.7 per cent) in the proportion allocated to health in this period by the developed countries (World Bank 1985).

At a second level, resource constraints have been made worse within the health sector by financial allocations which do not sustain primary and preventive care. In Sri Lanka, 70 per cent of the state's recurrent health expenditure goes on curative services, and of the 25 per cent spent on preventive services over half is allocated to the vertical malaria campaign. Similarly, in Colombia, 80 per cent of the government's recurrent health budget goes to hospitals. The production of health personnel is heavily in favour of the most expensive cadre: there are 23,000 doctors in the country, with only 6,000 professional nurses and 26,000 auxiliary nurses. Most of the doctors live in the cities. In Botswana, a new hospital was opened in Francistown in 1987, and work began on upgrading the main referral hospital in Gaborone. Additional recurrent expenditure and staff allocations will be required to support these tertiary facilities, possibly at the expense of primary facilities. This picture is repeated throughout the developing world: in general, 50–60 per cent of all government health spending in many countries is directed towards the provision of urban-based hospital care (Mills 1987).

The final problem is that, within this allocation pattern, resources are used inefficiently. Buildings are constructed without ensuring that adequate numbers of personnel – or supplies of drugs – will be available. This results in the provision of only a limited range of poor-quality care. Existing buildings are left to deteriorate rather than being regularly maintained. Malawi's major referral hospital, for example, has identified potential savings within its recurrent budget of nearly 33 per cent of the total budget (Government of Malawi 1986). Within drug distribution and supply systems, economies can vary from an average of 10 per cent through better drug selection to 45 per cent as a result of improved drug storage and distribution (WHO 1989).

But it is difficult to make such savings, and they are not achieved quickly. Changing the pattern of allocations is even harder and would require challenging the political pressures brought by urban populations, wealthy elites and specialist doctors. Being the lowest-level health worker in the hierarchy, CHWs have least voice, and are therefore the easiest cadre to trim or forget when budgets are tight.

Community support for community health worker programmes

Many governments have looked to communities for support for CHW programmes, often giving as a rationale that in this way communities will control the performance of their CHWs as the CHWs will be accountable to them. As we have seen, most experience suggests that communities are relatively passive and in fact exert very little control over their CHWs – who tend to identify most closely with the health system rather than with the community. Only a few instances exist where communities hold the purse strings and pay CHWs from, for example, drug sales (Jancloes 1985).

Whichever theoretical rationale governments have put forward for involving the community in support of CHWs, it appears that they have only seen this option in a very limited way. Abel-Smith and Dua (1988) suggest that community financing is often seen as 'contributions by individual or family beneficiaries or community groups to support a part of the cost of the health services', and that a fuller description should be 'collective action – a concerted action for the benefit of people who share a common interest or purpose'. The first definition focuses on the financing side of the concept – financially sustaining health programmes. The other emphasizes the community involvement side of the concept, in which it is the collective action (financial or otherwise) that sustains the enterprise. Governments have generally been more interested in shedding some of the costs of CHWs and other health activities than in mobilizing communities' participation in health programmes. In any case, it is difficult to impose participation or to enforce mobilization nationally. Community financing of the second definition requires quite different strategies and processes than those used in planning national CHW programmes.

What form has community support for community health workers taken?
We have seen that community support for CHWs may, for example, be by
the community members building health facilities for the CHWs;
alternatively, they could pay them directly (in cash or kind), or indirectly. It
is rare for such projects to have been without problems. One review of over
100 projects concluded:

> The most common forms of community support are voluntary labour
> and direct personal payments, and both have limited utility. Voluntary
> labour is useful chiefly for one-time construction costs, while direct
> personal payments place the financing burden on the sick and limit
> access to persons who can afford to pay. Community financing, at
> best, is just one element of a balanced financing approach. It has not
> paid for supervision, logistical support or referral linkages and can be
> effective only if these services are financed from other sources (APHA
> 1982).

In 1985 a study sponsored by the Christian Medical Commission looked
into the possibility of PHC programmes becoming self-reliant through
communities' paying for services. They analysed a number of Church-
supported programmes in Indonesia, the Philippines, Papua New Guinea,
India and Brazil, and concluded that, while individuals were sometimes
willing to pay for well-organized curative services, this seldom applied to
preventive services. Furthermore, well run programmes

> have a tendency to grow both in volume of services and number of
> locations served. Although they may be intrinsically heading for a
> degree of self-reliance, their very 'success' means that they will need
> additional funding, thus disturbing the strategy of phasing out outside
> support (Christian Medical Commission 1987).

The report added that not only were PHC programmes unlikely to become
financially self-supporting, but where communities were asked to pay for
some of their services there were real dangers that the poorest groups would
not be able to afford such services.

Harnmeijer (1988) has calculated that if each Zambian CHW were to
receive an allowance of 20 kwacha (US $3.00) per month, and assuming the
catchment population per CHW to be fifty households, the cost of the
allowance would be the equivalent of just over 1 per cent of the average
annual household income. Although this appears a small amount it is still
unclear what burden it would represent for those with below-average
incomes, and it 'could be prohibitive in the absolute sense when basic food
is often not guaranteed or available' (Harnmeijer 1988). Other demands on
household income also have to be considered: what priority is given to
clothing, soap and household essentials, to contributions for education or
the water supply, relative to health expenditure? Similar concerns have been
raised in the debate about whether to charge fees for health care (Gilson
1988).

Although experience has shown that community members are prepared to pay for some services, willingness to pay depends on a number of factors: perceptions of the value of the service being offered; the existence of alternative sources of the same or similar service; and people's economic security. How do these affect the likelihood of communities' paying for CHWs? Given the few curative skills that CHWs have, is it likely that they will be valued (and therefore supported) by the community? If the cost is relatively low, and the benefit of incurring that cost is considered high (such as receiving antibiotics or pain relievers), then people may be willing to pay. If, on the other hand, the cost is high and the perceived benefit low (as in the building of a latrine), then the chances of paying for it are extremely low.

Where communities, rather than government or non-governmental organizations, have been expected to pay for CHWs, the consequences for programme sustainability have been very mixed, and largely negative. For example, high attrition rates among community health agents in Ethiopia were explained by the fact that remuneration was irregular or non-existent, in spite of clear mechanisms through which it should have been paid: peasant associations, service co-operatives and producers' co-operatives. The two latter types of organization, more highly developed than the peasant associations which consisted of individual farmers, were more likely to remunerate community health agents through the sale of drugs, but even they failed to do so more often than not (Meche *et al.* 1984). In some programmes, CHWs support themselves through charging for consultations or medicines, sometimes at levels agreed by community institutions. This may be sufficient to keep CHWs working if they have a regular supply of drugs, or if there are no other cheaper sources of drugs. In some countries drugs are easily available, even in quite remote rural areas, and the limited supplies that CHWs are allowed may not be what is wanted by the population. For example, some villagers in projects in both Mali and Senegal were willing to purchase basic drugs from CHWs, but in both cases the per capita expenditure on drugs was a fraction of what had been expected given the population and disease profile (Gray 1986).

Experience suggests two lessons: communities are poor, and they will only pay for services that are of value at that particular time. Traditional midwives usually receive some sort of gratitude in cash or kind straight after the delivery. Villagers will find payment for treatment or drugs when they are ill. But where CHWs have mainly an educative role, villagers are not usually prepared to remunerate them. For example, in Swaziland, even when a form of payment was devised whereby communal land and labour was designated in order to pay the health motivators, the scheme did not achieve fruition (Connolly and Dunn 1986). A major problem in sustaining CHWs through community financing, therefore, is that often they are not highly valued.

Building confidence in CHWs is all-important. A government CHW programme in Somalia, strongly backed by Unicef, used two ways of ensuring support for CHWs: first, the programme was regularly supplied with drugs and supervision; and second, much effort went into talking to communities about how they could remunerate their CHWs, and importantly, no attempt was made either to impose a method or to make it uniform. Thus each community produced its own solution. Gradually payments in kind (cigarettes, sugar, rent-free accommodation) were replaced with longer-lasting, more viable alternatives. For example, one community instituted a tax on the village water pump: from the takings it was possible to pay a CHW and a watchman, as well as to buy pump spares and lubricants. Another village waived fees for water rights for the CHW's family. Larger villages found that a levy on tea-shops was both convenient and good for public relations. In nomadic communities it was easier to pay with livestock once a year, after herds had survived the dry season (Bentley 1989).

There is little doubt that this programme was successful because of the way it was implemented, and the technical assistance and financial inputs from Unicef cannot be underestimated. Indeed, Bentley (1989) says that although local-level efforts were successful, it proved much more difficult to train and motivate middle-level ministry of health staff. Without the Unicef inputs, would the programme continue to work successfully?

Unpaid volunteers

An alternative way of sharing the cost of CHWs with the community is to introduce a volunteer cadre. In reality, of course, it is not the community that bears the cost burden of volunteers, but the volunteers themselves, and their families.

Sri Lanka is one of a number of countries that have had large volunteer health programmes since the mid-1970s. Indonesia, Burma and Thailand have all trained part-time health workers on a large scale. It is unlikely that such programmes would be possible in all situations, and it is interesting to look at the characteristics of these societies to understand how they have been able to sustain large volunteer programmes, even with high attrition rates.

For at least two of the countries an important condition seems to be that there are large numbers of relatively well-educated young people with few job opportunities. Another enabling factor may be a religious or cultural ethos that encourages voluntarism. Buddhism is the main religion in Burma, Thailand and Sri Lanka. In Indonesia a strong authoritarianism encourages participation at village level.

These examples are all of large rural programmes. In Botswana, where there are few educated young people in the rural areas, conventional wisdom has suggested that voluntarism in health activities is unlikely. Many years of drought relief with 'food for work' schemes have resulted in expectations of payment for work performed. In Colombia some volunteer projects have been started in urban areas, but only on a small scale, and relatively recently, making it difficult to assess their sustainability.

Common problems of volunteer programmes are that they cannot expect people to work full-time, and because of the voluntary nature of the work it is difficult to control the quality and amount of work done. Skills are therefore largely educational, which may both limit effectiveness and the interest for the volunteer. It is relatively unusual for part-timers to be given curative skills. The viability of voluntary programmes depends to an even greater extent than salaried programmes on good support and regular contact: incentives may be simple, but they need to be built in. In general, attrition rates from voluntary programmes are high, although, as we have seen with Sri Lanka, this need not be seen negatively if it is assumed that one of the goals of the volunteer programme is mass community health education.

Most CHWs, however, are paid. A review of twenty-six different Oxfam projects showed that only four did not pay their health workers, and concluded that without external assistance and support CHW schemes would probably fail (Walt 1986). Indeed, an evaluation of Oxfam projects in India observed that when Oxfam's active support was withdrawn, CHW schemes came to a standstill (Ramprasad 1985).

Sharing the burden of sustaining community health worker programmes

Community support for CHW programmes has often, as discussed, been promoted by governments in order to ease their burden of sustaining the programmes. Although it is unclear how this burden has been shared within communities, it appears that the cost has not been allocated fairly between them. Usually it is the areas least provided with other forms of health care that have been expected to sustain CHW programmes, while government resources have continued to be channelled to the more privileged communities. However, it has also been argued that community financing has either promoted or preserved equity because it has improved the accessibility of services to previously underserved areas, and because communities have generally been willing to adjust financial demands for those considered 'indigent':

> While it was, of course, inequitable that communities in these cases had to pay for care that others got for free, the new services that community financing made possible resulted in a net contribution to the public welfare (Stinson 1987).

Judging whether the burden of sustaining CHW programmes has been fairly allocated is not easy, but it is important. For it is not enough that CHWs should be sustained, but that this should be achieved in a manner compatible with the PHC approach – which is rooted in a concern for social justice, emphasizing equity and community participation (Gilson 1989).

Sustainability requires more than financing

From his review of many community financing projects, Stinson (1987) concludes that sustainability is a complex problem that does not depend only on increased resource generation. More effective planning, to both respond to – and shape – demand, is also important, as is improving the quality of services by increasing worker stability and performance, and strengthening fiscal accountability.

The experience of CHW programmes suggests both that the problem of ensuring their sustainability has all too often been forgotten and that, where it has been considered, has simply been seen as an issue of paying the CHWs. Costs have not been adequately assessed during the planning stages of programmes, while the possible contributions of existing services – and the limits on those contributions – have been forgotten, and 'the community' has been viewed as the final back-up for programmes. Instead of considering the sustainability of CHW programmes in the context of the sustainability of all health-sector activities, the burden of support has been laid at the door of those perhaps least able to deal with it – the rural populations. Moreover, the section of the health services closest to these populations, and to the CHWs, is itself stretched to breaking point, as resource shortages and inefficient resource use, undermine the support required to guarantee continuity of care at the primary level. Small wonder that so many CHW programmes have faltered. Those calling for the complex solutions required to ensure the sustainability of the programmes have been drowned out by the demands of the urban populations – and many in the medical profession – to protect the high-technology and urban-based services.

References

Abel-Smith, B. and Dua, A. (1988). Community financing in developing countries: the potential for the health sector. *Health Policy and Planning*, 3, 2, 95–108.

APHA (1982). *Community Financing of Health Care*. American Public Health Association, Washington, DC.

Bentley, C. (1989). Primary health care in northwestern Somalia: a case study. *Social Science and Medicine*, 28, 10, 1019–30.

Berman, P. (1984). Village health workers in Java, Indonesia: coverage and equity. *Social Science and Medicine*, 19, 4, 411–22.

Berman, P., Gwatkin, D. and Burger, S. (1987). Community-based health workers: head start or false start towards health for all? *Social Science and Medicine*, 25, 5, 443–59.

Chabot, J. and Waddington, C. (1987). Primary health care is not cheap: a case study from Guinea Bissau. *International Journal of Health Services*, 17, 3, 387–409.

Christian Medical Commission (1987). *Financing Primary Health Care Programmes*. Christian Medical Commission, Geneva.

Connolly, C. and Dunn, L. (1986). *Development of Appropriate Methods for Sustaining Rural Health Motivators*. Research Paper 20, University of Swaziland.

de Salazar, L. *et al*. (1987). Costos de unidades del primer nivel de atención. Unpublished mimeo, Centro de Investigaciones Multidisciplinarias en Desarrollo (CIMDER), Cali, Colombia.

de Savigny, D. *et al*. (1988). *Village Health Worker Training in Kilombero District: Cost Aspects*. CUAMM, Dar es Salaam.

Ennever, O. *et al*. (1988). The use of community health aides as perceived by their supervisors in Jamaica, East Indies (1987/88). *West Indies Medical Journal*, 37, 131–8.

Gilson, L. (1987). District planning management and resource allocation model: costs of services and infrastructure. Unpublished mimeo, London School of Hygiene and Tropical Medicine.

Gilson, L. (1988). *Government Health Care Charges: Is Equity Being Abandoned?* Publication no. 15, Evaluation and Planning Centre, London School of Hygiene and Tropical Medicine.

Gilson, L. (1989). Financing systems within PHC. In *Alma Ata: Ten Years After*. Royal Tropical Institute, Amsterdam.

Government of Malawi (1986). *The National Health of Malawi 1986–1995*. Lilongwe: Government Printers.

Gray, C. (1986). State-sponsored primary health care in Africa: the recurrent cost of performing miracles. *Social Science and Medicine*, 22, 3, 361–8.

Harnmeijer, J.W. (1988) Recurrent costs in primary health care: examined in relation to the national primary health care programme of the Republic of Zambia. Unpublished MSc dissertation, London School of Hygiene and Tropical Medicine/London School of Economics.

Harnmeijer, J.W. (1989). Personal communication.

Heaver, R. (1984). *Adapting the training and visit system for family planning, health and nutrition programmes*. Staff working paper no. 662, World Bank, Washington, DC.

Jancloes, M. (1985). Financing urban primary health care services. *Tropical Doctor*, 15, 2, 9–104.

Meche, H., Dibeya, T. and Bennett, J. (1984). The training and use of community health agents in Ethiopia. *Ethiopian Journal of Health Development*, 1, 1, 31–40.

Mills, A. (1987). *The Financing and Economics of Hospitals in Developing Countries*. World Bank PHN Technical Note Series no. 87–20. Washington, DC.

Over, M.A. (1986). The effect of scale on cost projections for a primary health care programme in a developing country. *Social Science and Medicine*, 22, 3, 351–60.

Ramprasad, V. (1985). *Critique of an Experience*. Report of the study on the community health programmes funded by Oxfam (India) Trust, Bangalore, India.

Stinson, W. (1987). *Creating Sustainable Community Health Projects: The Pricor Experience*. Chevy Chase, Maryland: Primary Health Care Operations Research.

Walt, G. (1986). *Village Health Workers in Some Oxfam Projects*. Oxfam Discussion Paper, 1. Health Unit, Oxfam, Oxford.

WHO (1988). *Health Economics: A Programme for Action*. Geneva: WHO.

WHO (1989). Financing of essential drugs. Report of a WHO Workshop, Geneva. Unpublished mimeo.

World Bank (1985). *World Development Report, 1985*. Oxford University Press, Oxford.

PART III
Case studies

6 | Evaluating community health worker programmes

By definition, community health workers (CHWs) are the least accessible health workers, with informal or minimal ties to institutional health services. Both logistically and methodologically, evaluations of CHW programmes are fraught with difficulties.

Because of logistic constraints, CHWs are difficult to assess. Observation may be the only way to ascertain what they are doing, how much time they spend on assigned tasks, and how well they do them. Even if evaluators were to have time to observe CHWs on a day-to-day basis, methodological difficulties abound. For example, the very presence of researchers may affect how the CHWs work. Such research is time-consuming and expensive if it is to cover sufficient numbers of CHWs to draw general conclusions.

Besides financial and time costs, there may be a reluctance to evaluate CHW schemes where they are being supported, wholly or partly, by external funding, because of the fear of a critical outcome and withdrawal of funds. Alternatively, donor interests may coincide with government interests and may accentuate the positive side of programmes, despite little real evidence to support their claims. Any programme supported by foreign aid is subject to pressures for increased extension and an appearance of achievement.

In this chapter we first describe the research process used in the study that forms the basis for this book. We then look at some of the theoretical and methodological problems of evaluating CHW programmes in general. Finally, we describe the guidelines we used as a basic framework for the whole study.

The research process

As explained in the Preface, this book is the result of a study which set out to re-examine the implementation of national CHW programmes, looking at the policy, planning and management implications of this experience. The research process consisted of reviewing existing material on CHW programmes from all over the world, and then undertaking, with national research partners, three in-depth country case studies.

Before the country case studies were chosen, published and unpublished information on CHWs was collected from as many sources as possible, through contacts with international and aid agencies, non-governmental organizations, universities, and so on. This review was followed by interviews with policy-makers in international and non-governmental agencies who were themselves involved in CHW programmes. Through this process it was possible to build up a realistic picture of CHW programmes and to begin to identify those countries with established national programmes in which in-depth collaborative studies could be carried out.

As each case study was unique in itself, it was decided to choose countries from different regions of the world (Asia, Africa and Latin America). The main criteria for choosing countries were that they currently operated CHW programmes which had been in existence for at least ten years, that they were part of national government – or ministry of health – policy, and that they were not confined just to small parts of the country. Exploratory information was collected from seventeen countries, from which six (two in each of the three regions) were identified as potential collaborators. In March and April 1986 each Evaluation and Planning Centre (EPC) team member of the London School of Hygiene and Tropical Medicine visited four of these countries to explore the in-country support for – and feasibility of – a collaborative research project. The aim was to identify one or two individuals who would be the main collaborators within a suitable co-ordinating institution. The three countries with which collaboration was ultimately established were Botswana, Colombia and Sri Lanka.

In each country the research was designed by a team that included the national researchers and two members of the EPC team. It took place at two levels: at the national level, exploring the evolution of health policy in relation to the CHW programme; and at a local level, where specific priorities and concerns of the country were addressed. The focus of each case study was, therefore, slightly different.

The national-level interviews and document review were carried out jointly where possible, but most of the local research was undertaken by the national research team. The EPC team returned to each country after the main research had been done to help in the analysis and writing-up of the country study. Meetings were held at national level to feed back the findings of the study, and to discuss conclusions and recommendations with national policy-makers concerned with the CHW programme.

The process of disseminating the main research findings culminated in an international workshop in London in 1988, when the central collaborators from each country and the EPC team reported on the studies. The workshop participants were invited because of their experience and knowledge of CHW programmes. They took part in a discussion about the future of CHW programmes and the options facing national policy-makers. This book is the final part of the dissemination process.

Before attempting to explore national CHW programmes in the three countries chosen for in-depth study, we had to consider the methodological problems involved in evaluating CHW programmes. In the following section we briefly discuss some of these issues.

Methodological issues

Rigorous evaluations of CHW programmes are difficult to undertake, largely because there are enormous methodological problems both in research design and logistics. This does not mean that it is impossible to assess a CHW programme, rather that there are many limitations that have to be taken into account.

In a sense, the best possible evaluation is to be able to show whether a programme had an *impact* on the health of the community it was serving. Thus the aim would be to demonstrate that, after introducing CHWs to a certain community, health improved. This could be shown by a fall in infant mortality, for example, or a clear reduction in the number of deaths from measles. However, while the effectiveness of a CHW programme might best be assessed by changes in mortality and disease prevalence in the community, it is notoriously difficult to design evaluations that can confidently demonstrate causal relationships between CHW inputs and decreases in mortality or morbidity. Separating the influence of CHWs from any other influences on health status is almost impossible. Thus measuring impact is not an evaluation methodology usually attempted for CHW programmes. The few examples that exist are of special, small programmes and – even with these, CHW inputs could not be separated from other primary health care (PHC) inputs (Berggren *et al*. 1981). It should be said that measuring the influence of other health workers, such as doctors or nurses, on the health of a country's citizens is equally difficult and seldom attempted.

Measuring *outcomes*, such as changes in nutrition, provision of malaria prophylaxis, or the percentage of children immunized, is sometimes undertaken. However, there are again limitations to what can be quantified. A careful evaluation needs fairly large numbers and matched control populations – which are not always easy to find. Separating the influence of CHWs from others with whom they work is rarely possible. Measuring such outcomes depends on base-line studies, on records being available and/or on observational visits. Although records often exist for immunizations (through health services or child growth charts), other CHW records are usually simple and are often incomplete and inaccurate. Visits for observation are time-consuming and carry the risk of observation bias, especially if they have been arranged in advance. Furthermore, since most

CHW tasks are preventive, promotive or educational, an estimate of their efficiency should reflect these skills in changing behaviour as well as knowledge and attitudes. For example, CHWs may increase mothers' knowledge about when to use oral rehydration salts and how to mix them, but this does not necessarily mean that the mothers will actually use oral rehydration when children have diarrhoea. Assessing CHWs' influence in changing behaviour thus does not lend itself to easy quantitative assessment. Only a few evaluations of small-scale programmes have attempted to measure the effect of CHWs' inputs on behaviour related to immunization or antenatal care (Bhattacharji *et al.* 1986).

Monitoring the *outputs* of CHW schemes is what many evaluations attempt. Evaluators may count the number of home visits made by CHWs, or health education talks they have given. They may look at the opportunities CHWs have for attending continuing education courses, how often supervisory support is provided, and so on (Meche *et al.* 1984; Enge *et al.* 1984; Marchione 1984; Bentley 1989). Such evaluations will depend on the availability of routine information, and on some record of activities or courses held. Where records do not exist, evaluators have to rely on memory, which can be less reliable.

Some evaluations attempt to measure the quality of outputs. For example, they may try to assess what happened during the supervisory visit: was it merely to check the CHW's supplies and records, or was it an occasion used to discuss problems, or to reinforce knowledge? Although this sort of information is clearly most reliable if collected by observation during the supervisory encounter, evaluators often have to rely on questioning the health workers themselves about what happened. Clearly claims or memories may not be accurate. Similarly, many evaluations include questions about the perceptions that professional staff and communities have of CHWs and their work, and sometimes they include the perceptions and attitudes of the CHWs themselves (Maru 1983). While the answers to these questions can be valuable tools for identifying weaknesses in programmes, they are not always reliable, and they are seldom able to give any real indication of the quality of such encounters.

Other evaluations attempt to assess the extent to which CHWs have increased equity, by providing access to services to a wider number of people than before (Berman 1984). One way is to identify who in the community is served by the CHW: is it largely the rich, or the poor? Women or men? Are community members using primary health services more (because of CHW referrals) or less (because CHWs provide a satisfactory service nearer to home)? Obtaining reliable answers to such questions needs extremely careful research design and methods.

It is not only the actual methods used for evaluation which have to be considered. There are many other questions which must be addressed before an evaluation is carried out, and which help focus on the reasons why the evaluation is taking place.

The evaluation process

A number of simple questions help focus the process:

why, who, where, what and how?

Why evaluate?

Although evaluations ought to be for health workers as well as for policy-makers, the former are seldom involved in evaluation as a process of monitoring. The focus in many evaluations, rather, is more on accountability to donors or ministry of health officials than on programme and staff development. Thus an evaluation is often initiated externally (by a donor, for example), to satisfy the donor's constituency: either to show how public contributions of money can assist development in poor countries, or to assess whether programmes should continue to be supported. The ministry of health, which is usually involved in donor evaluations (see, for example, Government of Somalia/Unicef 1986), will often justify such an evaluation as being a useful way of informing officials of how a programme is being implemented, and of highlighting its weaknesses. The extent to which action is taken once recommendations have been made depends on many things, not least the extent to which the evaluation was imposed on, or initiated by, the ministry of health. Some evaluations have been undertaken by national academic institutions, sometimes supported financially by donors (see, for example, Hongvivatana *et al.* 1987). These may or may not attract the attention of policy-makers in the ministry of health. Our experience suggests that evaluations would be much more useful if all health staff were involved, not in one-off evaluations, but as part of an ongoing process of monitoring.

Who conducts the evaluation?

Evaluations are often done by outside experts, who may or may not be foreigners. Such evaluators can be useful since they may bring a new approach to a programme, or may be able to be more open or critical than those who are directly involved. However, our research suggests that the people who *should* be involved in evaluations are in fact the supervisors of CHWs, because very often they know little about the work of their CHWs. To put this into practice, in any CHW programme supervisors could spend two or three days each month with a group of CHWs, living with them in their villages, so that supervisory visits could be much more than the usual one or two hours spent every few months. This is the only way to gauge the quality of the CHWs' work and to discover the factors that may be inhibiting their effectiveness. All supervisors should be armed both with checklists for supervision – that include some notion of the quality of community encounters or interventions – and with skills to hold group discussions and interviews with key informants in the community. The contact between supervisor and CHW should be part of the CHWs' continuing education.

Where should attention be focused in local evaluation processes?

Conventionally, most evaluations start by examining the objectives of the programme and assessing how far these have been met. An evaluation may, for example, concentrate on the extent to which CHW programmes have extended PHC services to neglected areas (Owuor-Omondi et al. 1986). However, evaluations have revealed surprisingly little information about the activities in which CHWs are actually involved, how much time they spend on tasks, or the costs involved in the CHW programme. Such information is difficult to collect in a one-off evaluation, and our experience suggests that more attention should be focused on local activities as part of the monitoring process.

It is supervisors who need to look at CHW activities with a critical eye and, in discussion with CHWs, to weigh up the advantages and disadvantages of carrying out particular functions. Setting priorities, in terms of time, activities and target groups, is likely to lead to better-quality care if there is agreement and understanding about what is being listed. Supervisors need training in communicating with CHWs and in the simple techniques each of them can use to measure progress.

What is to be evaluated?

As is made clear in the discussion on methodology, most evaluations are concerned with processes. A clear focus should be on quality, although target outcomes should also be set as goals for CHWs to reach – as ways in which progress and change can be measured. The style the supervisor takes with the CHW should be as democratic and discursive as possible, leading through discussion to decisions, rather than the autocratic or bureaucratic style often adopted by professionals towards others lower in the hierarchy.

How are evaluations carried out?

This depends on what records are kept, the time available, how dispersed the communities are, training in evaluation methods, interest and motivation. Many methods can be used, both qualitative and quantitative, such as

- questionnaires, either self-administered or completed by trained researchers;
- focus-group discussions with CHWs, health professionals, community members;
- household surveys by trained researchers;

- perusal of records;
- in-depth interviews;
- inventories of equipment, drugs and supplies.

In general, using a combination of these methods will obtain more helpful information for the same investment than if only one method is employed. For example, a large evaluation of the Indian CHW programme used questionnaires to ask community members how much they valued their CHWs. Ninety per cent of those questioned said they were satisfied with the services of the CHW, and the evaluation concluded that the CHWs were serving all socio-economic strata (Maru 1983). However, other evaluations of the Indian scheme have cast doubt on these findings (Quadeer 1985). It is possible that questionnaires evoke answers the communities think the evaluators want to hear, and that had group discussions been held, the evaluation may have been more cautious in its interpretation of community satisfaction.

Although it is common to find many different statistics and forms being completed at primary-level health facilities, staff are seldom aware of their epidemiological value, and our research underlined this. An ongoing evaluation process could make much more use of quantitative methods to help staff and CHWs monitor their own activities. Although randomly sampled household surveys are probably only occasionally possible, and may need external assistance to execute, useful information can be obtained for example, by making selected visits to households which have recently received a home visit and to those which have not and drawing relevant comparisons. In addition, all peripheral health workers, including CHWs, should know approximately how many households they are supposed to cover (census data and maps are often available), and how to do simple studies. One example would be a study to see which families have attended preventive clinics (clinics often routinely record addresses of attenders) in order to identify those who have not attended so that they can be given special attention.

All primary health workers (including CHWs) should have some idea of the size of their target populations, such as numbers of children under three years, numbers of women in the fertile age groups, and numbers of disabled, tuberculosis or leprosy patients. Inventories of the CHWs' equipment, drugs and supplies can reveal important shortages of vital items, or an excess of other items. Such quantitative information – which is of great value to both the health workers and their supervisors in assessing performance – can be obtained relatively simply, either by special studies or, preferably, as a routine part of the self-evaluation process.

Qualitative evaluation methods can also be of enormous value and should be used in conjunction with quantitative methods. Holding group discussions which focus on specific points and are designed to generate free discussion (by involving people of similar status and age, for example) can produce surprising information regarding habits, customs and attitudes.

Such sessions need trained facilitators who can lead the discussion in a non-judgemental and non-directional way, a skill that needs to be taught and cannot be assumed. Combining questionnaires with focus-group discussions can be a useful way of verifying statements. Such focus groups can be held with community members, to check their attitudes to – and expectations of – CHWs. They can also be held with groups of CHWs or health professionals, for similar reasons. Using self-administered questionnaires, and checking preferences against records where possible, gaps between intention or stated preference and actual performance can be identified.

Participant observation – unobtrusively taking part in an activity while observing the interactions and performance of others – can also give useful insights. Interviewing key informants, or a range of people providing or receiving a service, can also be valuable in building up a picture of what is happening. To do this, the evaluators need to spend some time *in situ*, but this need not be more than a few days (Scrimshaw and Hurtado 1987).

It is striking that although several evaluations of either CHW performance or CHW programmes have been carried out (for a review see Walt 1988), little can be concluded from their findings about the effectiveness of CHWs. This is partly due to the methodological difficulties already explored, and the financial implications of rigorous evaluation designs. In setting out to do a research study on CHW programmes we were aware of three major areas of weakness in past evaluations.

First, many evaluations undertaken over the past decade were initiated by external agencies with special interests in CHW programmes (sometimes because they had funded part of the programme). However, in most ministries CHW programmes take a relatively low position on the health-policy agenda. Evaluation reports therefore tend to sit on shelves and rarely lead to anything other than minor policy changes. The first objective, it seemed to us, was to ensure that any evaluation met the specific needs of the country in question, and tried to address problems identified by those involved in the programme.

Second, most past evaluations have focused only on the implementation of the CHW programme, and have not considered its costs within the whole PHC system, or the consistency of CHW policy with overall health-sector policies. By neglecting trends in financing, plans for manpower development and other issues high on the policy agenda, such evaluations have tended to produce conclusions and recommendations that do not present policy-makers with realistic options for change. We felt it important that any evaluation should consider the context within which CHW policy had been formulated and the programme implemented.

Third, evaluations have seldom been used as part of a process of learning lessons from how well – or badly – a programme is functioning. Such monitoring would provide opportunities for improving management and performance by involving both health staff and CHWs in a continuing process of evaluation. We felt strongly that, as much as possible, staff should have a role in the evaluation, and recommended that small evaluations could be used as methods of supervision and support and as monitoring tools for health workers involved in providing services.

Evaluation takes – and needs – time. It is best done with the aim of staff development rather than simple accountability. Supervisors should be trained in process evaluation methods that aim to improve management techniques.

Evaluation guidelines

The guidelines which follow describe the methodologies that we used, at both the national and local level, to evaluate CHW programmes in Botswana, Colombia and Sri Lanka. In attempting to establish how effective CHWs are, it was necessary to understand how the policy evolved from the beginning, and the support it generated, as well as to try to assess how CHWs were functioning at community level.

There were, thus, two important stages to our evaluation: a national-level study and a local-level study. As is made clear in the country studies, each addressed somewhat different concerns. However, in carrying out the evaluation, the following framework guided each of the country case studies.

National-level evaluation

The evolution and development of policy was explored through three phases: problem recognition and policy conceptualization; formulation of the policy and the programme; and implementation of the policy at national and local level. Although these phases are not easily distinguishable in the policy-making process, it is useful to think of them separately for analytical purposes. The first two concentrate on the historical development of the policy to train CHWs: the way decisions arose, and the consequent planning process once the policy had been decided. The third phase addresses the implementation of policy: the way it was put into practice and how well CHWs are functioning in the community. The following questions guided the evaluation:

Problem recognition and policy conceptualization
The first step here was to find out how the CHW programme became part of the policy agenda.

How, and from where, did support for a CHW programme emerge?

• for example, through a pilot scheme, non-government project, community experiment? who were the instigators?

- through international influence?
- within the ministry of health or outside it? locally or nationally?
- were there antecedents to the current CHWs (for example, volunteers)?

What were the underlying philosophy and objectives of the CHW programme?

- what were the objectives of the programme? for example, to extend health services? to increase community self-reliance?
- how explicit were the objectives? were they written down anywhere?

What was the basis of support for the CHW programme?

- was there any explicit calculation and discussion of the likely costs and possible sources of financial support for the CHW programme?
- who were the main protagonists? was there strong support from any particular group or institution? was there any resistance?

Formulation of the policy and the programme
The second step was to analyse the process of decision, planning and programming:

Who decided and planned the CHW programme?

- at national level
- at regional or district level
- at local level

Who made decisions about

- financing the programme?
- tasks, selection and training?
- teaching materials and methods?
- supervision and support?

What was the role of

- the professional bodies (nursing, medical etc.)?
- the planning unit or health manpower unit in the ministry of health?
- universities, medical and nursing schools?
- other ministries (local government, planning, finance, community development)?
- aid agencies?

Have there been modifications to the programme since inception?

- how did these come about? who initiated them?

Implementation of the policy at national and local level
Tracing the links between the different authorities involved in the CHW programme's implementation, and their specific role in its implementation,

was important because there were often several authorities involved, sometimes with diverse views of the part they should play. We asked

Who is responsible for implementing the CHW programme? (in terms of selection, training, supervision and support, payment, etc.)

- at the national level
- at regional or district level
- at local level

What is the role of

- the regional or district ministry of health officials?
- local-level nurses and doctors?
- other ministries?
- local authorities?
- communities?
- donors?

Is there co-operation between the various implementing agencies and individuals?

Methods used in evaluation

Several methods were used at each stage of the research, although their exact nature differed from one stage to the next. For the first two stages (which dealt with policy formulation), the main methods of evaluation were: interviews with key informants; examination of planning documents (policy statements, committee reports, national statistics, annual reports); and reviewing local journals, newspapers, professional papers. For the third stage (implementation), these same methods were used at the local level, together with special studies to ascertain how well CHWs were functioning both in terms of objective criteria (such as the balance of their different activities, the number of each of these carried out, their quality, the potential effect on the health of the target population, and their cost), and subjective criteria (such as the job satisfaction of the CHWs and the level of their appreciation by their colleagues, supervisors, the local community members and their leaders).

Community-level evaluation

At the community level, the broad question we asked was how well the CHWs were functioning. Were they

- achieving what is expected of them?
- contributing to extended coverage of health services, preventive and curative?
- forging links between the community and health service?

- improving the self-reliance of the community?
- acting as mechanisms for community participation?

The two central concerns of community-level studies are:

- *activities*: what do CHWs actually do, the extent to which their services are used, and the relationship between the CHWs' activities and the rest of the PHC system. This includes supervision, continuing education, provision of supplies, and so on.
- *perceptions*: of the community members, of the CHWs themselves, of other health workers – including motivation, satisfaction, the links and relationship between the community, the CHW and the rest of the health service.

Some important questions to ask of CHWs range around questions of activities, costs, community perceptions, CHW perceptions, health-worker perceptions and perceptions of community-based workers from other sectors:

Activities
What range of activities are they involved in?

How much time do they spend on preventive versus curative activities?

How much time do they spend home visiting and within health facilities?

How many homes do they visit per day or per week?

How many patients do they see per week in a facility?

What do they do during a home visit?

Do they intentionally or unintentionally target their activities towards certain subgroups of the population (for example, mothers and children, the rich or the poor, at-risk families, and so on)?

Do they modify their activities depending on the specific nature of the family they are dealing with, or give a standard 'package'?

What are they not allowed to do, officially or unofficially?

Who supervises them? How often do they receive supervision? What is done during a supervisory session? Do they receive any in-service training? (What kind? How often?) Do they receive adequate supplies?

Costs
Who pays for the CHW programme?

How much does it cost annually to run the CHW programme? How much per contact?

How many CHWs are there in the country? How many are actively working?

How long is their basic training? Where is it held? Who teaches the course?

What are the wage levels of the CHWs, their trainers, their supervisors, and others who support their work?

What drugs and other supplies do they use? How often are they supervised? By whom? From where? How many days (if any) of in-service training do they receive?

Community perceptions of the CHW
How do members of the community see their CHWs? Are they satisfied with them?

Are there important differences between the perceptions of different subgroups of the population (for example, by socio-economic status, ethnic group, age, sex?)

Which of their services do they most value?

What would they like the CHWs to do in addition or instead of current activities? Do they know what CHWs can do?

CHWs' perceptions
What issues do the CHWs identify as inhibiting the performance of their jobs?

Do they see themselves first as health workers or as community representatives?

Are they satisfied in their work? If not, why not?

Other health workers' perceptions
How do other local-level health workers see the CHWs?

Do they understand what the CHWs are supposed to do?

Do they value their activities? Are they supportive of CHWs in their activities?

Other sectors' workers' perceptions of the CHWs
How do other local-level community-based workers see the CHWs? Do they understand the role of the CHWs?

Do they collaborate with the CHWs? Why, and how?

These guidelines formed the framework within which we assessed the CHW programmes in Botswana, Colombia and Sri Lanka. Although the same basic approach was taken in each country, each case study addressed different concerns. In Botswana the main issue was the extent to which family welfare educators could become more community-orientated; in Colombia interest focused on methodological questions and programme performance; in Sri Lanka the central puzzle was to understand why CHWs volunteered. The detailed objectives of the research, and the methodology used, are described in each case study.

References

Bentley, C. (1989). Primary health care in northwestern Somalia: a case study. *Social Science and Medicine*, 28, 10, 1019–30.
Berggren, W.L., Ewbank, D.C. and Berggren, G.G. (1981). Reduction of mortality in rural Haiti through a primary health care program. *New England Journal of Medicine*, 304, 22, 1325–30.
Berman, P. (1984). Village health workers in Java, Indonesia: coverage and equity. *Social Science and Medicine*, 19, 4, 411–22.
Bhattacharji, S. *et al.* (1986). Evaluating community health worker performance in India. *Health Policy and Planning*, 1, 3, 232–9.
Enge, K. *et al.* (1984). *Evaluation: Health Promoter Program*. Ministry of Health, Lima. Management Sciences for Health, Boston, USA.
Government of Somalia/Unicef (1986). *Review of Primary Health Care 1986*. Ministry of Health, Somali Democratic Republic.
Hongvivatana, T. *et al.* (1987). *A Study of Alternatives to the PHC Volunteer and Community Organization Strategy*. Centre for Health Policy Studies, Mahihol University, Thailand.
Marchione, T. (1984). Evaluating primary health care and nutrition programmes in the context of national development. *Social Science and Medicine*, 19, 3, 225–35.
Maru, R. (1983). The community health volunteer scheme in India – an evaluation. *Social Science and Medicine*, 17, 19, 1477–83.
Meche, H., Dibeya, T. and Bennett, J. (1984). The training and use of community health agents in Ethiopia. *Ethiopian Journal of Health Development*, 1, 1, 31–40.
Owuor-Omondi, L., Atlholang, D. and Diseko, R. (1986). *The Changing Role of Family Welfare Educators?* National health status evaluation, Monograph series 1. Ministry of Health, Gaborone.
Quadeer, I. (1985). Social dynamics of health care: the CHW scheme in Shadol District. *Socialist Health Review* (September) 1, 74–83.
Scrimshaw, S. and Hurtado, E. (1987). *Rapid Assessment Procedures for Nutrition and Primary Care: Anthropological Approaches to Improving Program Effectiveness*. University of California, Los Angeles.
Walt, G. (1988). *Community Health Workers: Policy and Practice in National Programmes*. EPC Publication 16, London School of Hygiene and Tropical Medicine.

7 | Family welfare educators in Botswana

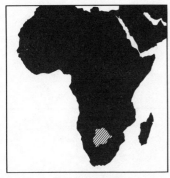

6 Map of Africa, with Botswana highlighted. Drawn by Geoff Penna.

The history of Botswana's community health workers (CHW) programme began in the late 1960s with a small pilot scheme for six mature women. Within four years, however, these CHWs, called family welfare educators (FWEs), had captured the interest of policy-makers to such an extent that the scheme was adopted as national policy. But in the transformation from a relatively small, flexible pilot project, the role of the FWE changed. Instead of being based largely in the community, and spending at least half their time on home-visiting, they rapidly became immersed in clinic work. Why did this occur? Was it a case of unrealistic expectations or poor planning? To understand what happened we have to view them in the context of health policy within their country.

Country background

The Republic of Botswana is a landlocked state lying in the centre of the Southern African Plateau. Slightly larger than France, two-thirds of the country is in the Kgalagadi desert. The country's geographical position generates a semi-arid continental climate. The annual average rainfall is about 475 mm, but it is erratic and unevenly distributed.

Most of the country's population is to be found along the fertile and relatively mild catchment area of the Limpopo river, in the eastern part of the country. The 1981 census found that total population was 941,027, growing rapidly at 3.5 per cent per year to reach an estimated 1,127,888 by

1986. As Table 6 shows, the population is a young one, reflecting both the high fertility and declining mortality rates. The infant mortality rate fell from 97 per 1,000 in 1971 to 71 per 1,000 in 1981, and to an estimated 65.3 per 1,000 in 1986. Although the population is largely concentrated in one part of the country, settlement is not dense (only 1.9 people per square kilometre in 1986) and the population is predominantly rural (only 21.7 per cent urban in 1986).

Table 6 Demographic indicators, Botswana.

		1981	1986 (estimated)
Enumerated population	Total	941,027	1,127,888
	Male	443,104	536,866
	Female	497,923	591,022
Population aged 0–4 (per cent)		19.4	20.1
Population aged 5–15 (per cent)		28.8	28.0
Sex ratio (males per 100 females)		89.0	90.8
Dependency ratio (per 100)		109.8	107.0
Crude birth rate (per 1000)		48.7	46.6
Crude death rate (per 1000)		13.9	12.6
Total fertility rate (births per woman)		7.1	6.9
Life expectancy at birth (years)	Males	52.3	53.5
	Females	59.7	60.6
Infant mortality rate (per 1000 births)		71.0	65.3

Source: National census, 1981

The economy

At the time of independence in 1966, Botswana was among the poorest countries in the world. Widespread poverty was entrenched after five years of serious drought, and over half the population was receiving food aid in 1966 (Egner and Klausen 1980). However, with large increases in mineral production since the early 1970s, Botswana's economy has experienced rapid growth and major structural changes. Per capita gross national product (GNP) rose, in current prices, from US $110 in 1970 to over US $900 in 1982, and gross domestic product (GDP) rose threefold between 1967 and 1978. In 1978 the World Bank removed Botswana from its list of the world's poorest countries and by 1986 it was categorized as a middle-income country with a per capita GNP of US $840.

The growth in mineral production, especially diamond mining, has led to a decline in the overall importance of agricultural production. Agriculture had been the major contributor to GDP in the early years of independence, but contributed only 12.2 per cent of GDP in 1980–1. The trading sector is also now more important to GDP than agriculture, contributing 23.9 per cent of GDP in 1980–1 (including revenues from the Southern Africa Customs Union). Major exports include diamonds, copper/nickel and beef.

The dualism of the economic structure, with a small productive formal sector and a large, relatively unproductive informal/subsistence agriculture sector, is reflected in the country's employment patterns. Although only a small proportion of the labour force is engaged in formal-sector employment (21.7 per cent in 1981), under- and unemployment in rural areas is estimated to be as high as 40 per cent. Employment in the South African mines used to be an important source of work but recruitment has declined by 54 per cent, from 40,390 in 1976 to 18,837 in 1987.

Income distribution patterns also reflect economic dualism. Despite remittances from household members working in urban areas or outside the country, the incomes of possibly one-half of the rural population indicate that they live in absolute poverty (Government of Botswana/Unicef 1986). The 1984 Rural Income Distribution Survey showed that the poorest 90 per cent received only 58 per cent of total rural income, while the richest 10 per cent received 42 per cent of total income. Similar skewed income distribution was found in a social and economic survey of peri-urban areas, which showed that the poorest 40 per cent of households received only 12 per cent of total income.

Botswana suffered a serious drought in the 1980s which has exacerbated such inequalities. Relief measures established by the government include drought-relief projects in many rural communities. For most people in these communities the projects have been their only source of household income. Supplementary food is also given to vulnerable groups including the destitute, chronic patients, pregnant mothers and children under five years of age. Such food-for-work and famine-relief projects may have eroded the fabric of voluntarism in Botswana. For example, one of the reasons given by village health committee members for their reluctance to volunteer their services is the feeling that they could utilize their time more productively by working on famine-relief projects (Owuor-Omondi et al. 1987).

Evolution of the political and administrative structure

Botswana attained independence from the British government on 30 July 1966, after one-and-a-half years of self-government. The laws of the country are made by a national assembly and general elections are held every five years. Below the national assembly is the house of chiefs which advises the government on matters relating to traditional customs and institutions.

There has been a gradual reduction of the powers of the chiefs with the decentralization of administrative authority since independence. The Local Government (District Councils) Bill (1965) first established district councils and empowered them, instead of the chiefs, to collect local taxes. These councils are now responsible for the administration, planning, implementation, monitoring and evaluation of development programmes in tribal areas. Below them are village-based institutions such as the village development committees (VDCs) which initiate development projects. Central government is linked to local authorities through the Ministry of Local Government and Lands (MLGL). Thus, the department of Unified Local Government Service (ULGS) within the MLGL appoints all appropriate staff required by district councils.

First created in 1974, as part of an expansion of central government, the Ministry of Health (MOH) is now decentralizing its administration of health services to fit in with the overall administrative structure.

Health and health services

The main health problems

Health problems in Botswana are similar to those of other developing countries, and have their roots in the economic conditions and climate. The relative importance of the main diseases has not changed much during the last ten years. Of the serious diseases, as judged by admission to hospitals, tuberculosis remains the most important and accounts for about 25 per cent of institutional deaths. Acute respiratory tract infections and diarrhoeal diseases account for 10 per cent of institutional deaths. These diseases particularly affect children; diarrhoeal diseases, for example, account for about 20 per cent of all recorded deaths in children under five years of age. Nutritional deficiencies statistically represent only 4 per cent of institutional deaths; however, the prevalence of undernutrition in children under five is almost 30 per cent and this contributes significantly to the incidence and effects of childhood infections.

Table 7 shows the leading causes of outpatient morbidity in 1984, as

Table 7 Leading causes of outpatient morbidity, Botswana, 1984.

	No of cases	%
Diseases of the respiratory system (excluding asthma)	497,819	28.5
Diseases of the digestive system	134,105	7.7
Diarrhoea	108,232	6.2
Gonorrhoea	75,635	4.3
Diseases of the skin and subcutaneous tissues	74,982	4.3
Accidents, injury, poisoning and violence (excluding burns and bites)	74,578	4.2
Diseases of the musculoskeletal system and connective tissue	72,192	4.1
Other diagnoses	712,108	40.7
TOTAL	1,749,651	100.0

Source: Ministry of Health (1984)

compiled from outpatient and preventive health statistics. The pattern of morbidity clearly reflects the mortality data, and is similar for all age groups. Thus, among the under-five age group, diseases of the respiratory system are the dominant cause of outpatient morbidity. However, as these are facility-based data they may not fully reflect the pattern of ill health in the community at large.

The health system

The MOH underwent a reorganization in 1984 following an organization and management review. The functions of the Ministry are now grouped into five major departments: PHC services; hospital services; technical support services; health manpower; and health administration. The national health research unit and the national health planning unit provide staff services to all departments and co-ordinate the specialist functions at national level.

The MOH, representing central government, has portfolio responsibility for the overall improvement of the health of the nation. As such, it sets the general goals, priorities and direction for the operation and development of health services and activities in Botswana. However, the basic health services are run by the local authorities, which comprise ten district councils and five town councils (all elected bodies) and which have statutory responsibility for the day-to-day operation of health posts and clinics. Within central government, the local authorities are also responsible to the MLGL for administrative matters.

In addition, medical missions and a number of large companies also provide health services, and complement the health-related activities of the MOH, other central government ministries, and the local authorities. The MOH, therefore, also has an important co-ordinating role to ensure that the whole health-care delivery system is operating efficiently, and that policies are understood and implemented by all the different agencies involved.

Since the 1970s, a PHC strategy has shaped the health services. About 85 per cent of the population now have reasonable access to health care, given the low density of settlement, and live within 15 km of a health facility. By 1984 the health system provided 375 mobile stops, 251 health posts, 128 clinics, 7 health centres and 15 hospitals. Regional health teams were set up by the MOH in 1974 to supervise and support the health services run by the local authorities, and these are functioning well. Indeed, to a great extent they can be held responsible for the success of the rural health services in Botswana. There are fairly uniformly high levels of utilization within the country – which are particularly encouraging given the very scattered nature of the population settlement pattern.

A move which it is hoped will contribute a great deal towards realizing community involvement is the recent policy to decentralize health services. The regional health teams will be placed operationally under district/town councils, and will be called district health teams. Through this move the MOH also hopes to strengthen the referral system.

Resources for the health services

The MOH's share of the total government expenditure has varied quite significantly over the years, falling to a low of 4.9 per cent in 1980 and rising to a high of 6.4 per cent in 1986. Such variation is basically due to changes in its share of development (capital) expenditure, which fell to 2.5 per cent of the government total in 1980 and has since risen to 6.4 per cent in 1986. By contrast, MOH recurrent expenditure has remained fairly constant, never falling below 7 per cent between 1979 and 1986.

Within the health sector overall, total expenditure in 1983–4 was estimated to be 56.4 million pula (14 million US $, 89 per cent recurrent, 11 per cent development), or 52.7 pula (13 million US $), per capita (Griffiths 1986). Roughly 61 per cent of recurrent expenditure was estimated to be funded from government sources (37 per cent MOH, 11 per cent local authorities and 13 per cent all other ministries), while out-of-pocket payments by individuals represented 20 per cent of the total. Non-governmental organizations (such as missions) funded 11 per cent, and industry 7 per cent. For development expenditure the MOH was the main channel of government funds (83 per cent of the total), although the 14 per cent contributed by local authorities was not insignificant.

These figures do not show the importance of either donor funding or traditional health care within the overall health sector. However, a study of health-sector expenditure in 1978–9 estimated official co-operation to be 10.9 million pula (2.75 million US $), more than the 8.9 million pula actually spent by the MOH. It was also estimated that individuals paid 3.3 million pula (0.8 million US $) to traditional healers, equivalent to 37 per cent of total MOH expenditure.

Perhaps the key non-financial health resource is personnel. Table 8 shows the 1984 personnel stock. Most health personnel are employed by government; and within government, most are employed either by the MOH or by the ULGS. Thus, 88 per cent of the total national nursing stock is employed by government – 53 per cent by the MOH and 35 per cent by the ULGS. FWEs are the lowest level of health personnel and 96 per cent are employed by the ULGS.

In terms of future resource availability for health care the key issue is the recurrent implication of existing development projects. Clearly, as secondary and tertiary facilities are expanded it is necessary to allocate additional recurrent funding to them. Failure to cover the additional recurrent needs, in particular, of the new Francistown hospital and the expanded Princess Marina hospital, will lead either to inadequate service provision from the new facilities, or to the withdrawal of resources from peripheral services to meet the demands of higher-level care. Current estimates suggest that, if past trends in budgetary increases are continued,

Table 8 Health personnel by category and employer, Botswana, 1984.

	Employer		
Category	Govt	Other[1]	Total
Doctors	109	47	156
Matrons	11	5	16
Senior sisters	32	8	40
Registered nurses/midwives	476	65	541
Family nurse practitioners	12	3	15
Community health nurses	20	0	20
Enrolled nurses-midwives	64	13	77
Enrolled nurses	726	104	830
Health inspectors	17	1	18
Health assistants	74	0	74
Family welfare educators	560	8	568
Total	2,101	254	2,355

[1] Mission, industry and private

Source: Ministry of Health (1984)

future MOH/local authority allocations may be insufficient to meet the new budgetary requirement of secondary and tertiary care.

The development of the family welfare educator programme

The first six FWEs were trained in 1969 by an expatriate doctor and a public health nurse who worked in Serowe council clinic in Central District. They were mature women whose previous work experience ranged from clinic cleaner to trained community development assistant. Funded by the International Planned Parenthood Federation (IPPF), their training was given on-the-job and focused on basic family planning with some maternal and child-health (MCH) care activities. Somewhat in conflict with this reality, the original goal of the programme was to train village women, selected by their own communities, as volunteer health workers – to be 'on the spot' in the village to help with common problems such as scabies, and to select those patients who most needed the regular visits of the doctor/nurse mobile team (Kromberg 1986). This goal was quickly overturned as the local authorities responsible for public health recognized the potential of using rapidly trained women to increase the existing very limited number of health staff for the rapidly expanding rural health services. Within a year of their first training course the FWEs were being paid, within two years they were an accepted national cadre, and by 1973 they had been transformed into local authority employees with uniforms, salaries and associated terms of service (Cook 1973; Bennett *et al.* 1980; Manyeneng 1982; Owuor-Omondi *et al.* 1986).

The historical growth of the rural infrastructure

These swift changes in the nature and number of FWEs occurred against the background of significant growth in the rural infrastructure of the country. As discussed above, Botswana was one of the poorest countries in Africa at independence in 1966 but by the early 1970s the economic situation had improved remarkably, and from 1972 government policy shifted towards rapid rural development. Several factors influenced this shift: the recurrent budget was balanced for the first time in 1972–3 and financial forecasts for surpluses in future years were optimistic; an election was due in 1974 about which the ruling Botswana Democratic Party (BDP) was purportedly nervous; and 83 per cent of the population lived in the rural areas (Colclough and McCarthy 1980); and a number of foreign aid agencies, notably NORAD of Norway and SIDA of Sweden, had expressed a preference for assisting rural rather than urban development. The accelerated rural development programme (ARDP) was launched in 1972–3 and there was considerable expansion of the rural infrastructure throughout the 1970s. During this period the economy grew rapidly, largely because of diamond mining.

Local institutions were also considerably strengthened at this time. Elected district councils superseded the pre-independence tribal authorities and were given statutory responsibilities in rural areas for primary education, public health services, sanitation, community development, public water supplies and roads, among other things (Egner 1987).

This general shift towards developing the rural infrastructure was also reflected in the health sector (Table 9). The previous highly centralized, hospital-orientated policies (Gish and Walker 1977) were transformed into PHC plans, with a strong emphasis on building rural health facilities – as was clearly reflected in the third National Development Plan (Government of Botswana 1972).

Table 9 Percentage allocation of development expenditure among health sector activities during the third National Development Plan, Botswana.

	1972–3	1974–5	1975–6	1976–7[1]
Hospitals	21.4	38.6	29.0	7.3
Health centres	5.1	3.1	10.2	2.9
Training	12.3	0.8	2.4	11.1
Rural health units	58.4	50.8	55.2	78.1
Other	2.8	6.7	3.2	0.6

[1] Estimated: there was a shortfall in spending of about 20%.

Source: Annual Statement of Accounts (annual report of the Ministry of Health), 1976.

The historical growth in education and training

Physical expansion had to be matched with manpower development. Primary school provision was the financial responsibility of the district and town councils, which devoted over half their recurrent expenditure to education during most of the years after 1966 (Colclough and McCarthy 1980). The proportion of children enrolled in primary schools almost doubled during the first thirteen years of independence (44 per cent of children were in primary school in 1965, 80 per cent in 1978), while secondary and tertiary levels increased sevenfold.

Training in the health sector also expanded during the 1970s. In 1969 there were 78 enrolled nurses, 250 registered nurses and 31 doctors in the country (including 4 private medical practitioners). By 1975 their numbers had risen to 269, 255 and 55, respectively, with even more rapid expansion in the following years (Table 10). The number of health staff had been supplemented by the new cadre of FWEs, of whom there were 154 by 1975. By then the greatest physical expansion of facilities had already occurred.

Table 10 Health facility and staffing changes, Botswana, 1970–84.[1]

	Hosp.	HC	Clinic	Health posts	Mobile stops	Doctors	Registered nurses[2]	Enrolled nurses	FWEs
1969	N/A	N/A	N/A	N/A	N/A	27	250	78	0
1975	14	7	58	N/A	208	55	255	269	154
1978	14	7	89	212	192	89	390	501	404
1982	15	7	123	239	389	142	548	791	560
1984	15	7	128	251	375	156	641	907	568

[1] Includes all known facilities and staff
[2] Includes all trained nursing staff, at every level of the health services
N/A = not available
Sources: Medical statistics annual reports, 1975–83; and Ministry of Health (1984)

The evolution of health policy

The policy climate that encouraged a rapid development of the rural infrastructure and an expansion of educational and training opportunities also fostered a rethinking in the health sector about the importance of primary health services. At the same time, the initial reluctance on the part of senior health officials to accept that FWEs could perform useful functions was challenged by growing demands for FWEs from district councils needing staff for new rural health posts. By 1974, a health facilities survey showed that Central District (where FWEs were first trained) had nineteen health posts staffed only by FWEs, and that there were a total of thirty-four such posts in the whole country.

This growing acceptance of the FWEs' potential role was reflected in the Department of Health Services' decision in 1973 to take over the administration and expenditure control of the annual IPPF training grant for FWEs (funding was later provided by Unicef). The Department also undertook to provide supervision and support when FWEs returned to their districts after training. Finally, together with the ULGS, the Department began to try to regularize the payment and conditions of service of FWEs, which until then had differed slightly from council to council. By 1974, when the Department of Health Services became a Ministry in its own right, FWEs were part of the established system of health services in Botswana.

In summary, the development of the FWE programme occurred at a time when government and donor policy was to expand and strengthen rural infrastructure and rural institutions. FWE training aided the opening of more health units. However, because this health facility expansion was the main force for training FWEs the original idea that they would be community based rapidly dissipated, and instead, they became associated with these facilities, helping to provide a variety of MCH-related services within them. The assumption that FWEs would spend half their time in the health units and half in the community thus never became a reality. In a number of excellent evaluations of the FWE programme (Cook 1973; Bennett et al. 1980; Manyeneng 1982; Owuor-Omondi et al. 1986) this has been the recurrent theme.

Methodology for this study

The evaluations mentioned above identified the major concern of policy-makers as the fact that the FWE was insufficiently community-orientated. Although some steps to reverse the bias towards clinic activities had been taken, such as curriculum revision, our study sought to identify clearly the overall feasibility of making the FWE less clinic-based and community-orientated. Its specific objectives were, first, to identify the factors that will facilitate or hinder the process of reorientating the FWEs towards a community-based approach; and second, to examine the practical feasibility of reorientating existing FWEs to such a community-based approach given different work settings (such as working alone or with others, with easy or poor access to supervisors).

Study methodology

Initially there were to be three study components: a national study, a study conducted by community health nurses (CHNs) and a study conducted by a researcher. However, in practice there was more involvement of the researcher and less involvement of the CHNs, because CHNs were not able to find the time to participate fully; they were, however, very helpful in facilitating contacts between the researcher and the community, and also in discussing preliminary findings with the researcher.

The main study components, therefore, were a national study and a district study. For the former, a questionnaire was sent to all the FWEs through the district medical officers, and also to all CHNs; a review of numerous FWE reports, evaluations and other relevant documents was undertaken; and interviews were conducted with relevant policy-makers and others in Gaborone. The latter study was undertaken by the researcher, in five districts: North-West, Francistown, Kweneng, Kgalagadi and South-East. At the community level the researcher where possible,

- administered questionnaires to village development committee (VDC) and village health committee (VHC) members;
- administered questionnaires to Red Cross officials;
- administered questionnaires to nurses at the local facility;
- conducted focus-group discussions with community members;
- accompanied each FWE on home visits, and recorded her observations about the visits; and
- analysed FWE home-visit record books.

At the district level the researcher

- administered individual questionnaires to district health team members;
- administered individual questionnaires to the district council chairman, secretary and matron; and
- conducted focus-group discussions with the district's FWEs.

Profile of the family welfare educator

There were estimated to be 609 FWEs working in Botswana in January 1987. A questionnaire was sent to them in that year, through the district health teams, and 553 forms (90.8 per cent) were returned to the MOH. Many of the findings from this questionnaire confirm those of previous small studies. What they emphasize is how far – in terms of selection, training, terms and conditions of work, and costs – the FWE programme has drifted from the original aims as envisaged by policy-makers.

A profile of the FWEs put together from this national questionnaire is shown in Table 11.

Table 11 Profile of family welfare educators, Botswana.

- 94% were female
- 56.2% were 30–39 years old
- 62.1% were single
- 39.4% had qualifications above the minimum level of standard 7 (7 years of schooling)
- 72.2% had over five years' experience as an FWE and 34.3% more than ten years' experience
- 82.6% worked in rural locations
- 23% worked in a health post by themselves

Source: National questionnaire, MOH–EPC, 1987

Selection, qualifications and transfers

In theory, FWEs should be selected by their communities, either through a *kgotla* (traditional community forum) or by the VDC or VHC. Candidates should be at least twenty years old, and should have completed primary school (seven years of schooling). Once they have returned to their community after training, it is expected that they will remain there for the duration of their working life as FWEs.

In fact, only 50.1 per cent were selected by the *kgotla*, VDC or VHC. All the others had applied directly to the local council for the position, or had been appointed. Selection by communities has been resisted by many councils over the years. As early as 1974 a circular from the establishment secretary of the ULGS remonstrated with councils for not following the official policies on selection, appointment and placement of FWEs. Owuor-Omondi *et al.* (1986) found that 45 per cent of FWEs had been appointed by members of the government health system.

In urban areas, town councils are under even greater pressure to appoint applicants, because the FWEs themselves argue that the communities are less stable and homogeneous. This practice was reflected in the finding that only two out of twenty-eight FWEs in Gaborone, and none of the twenty-six FWEs in Francistown (the two largest towns) had been selected either by *kgotla*, VDC or VHC. Moreover, 24 per cent had previously worked in a different facility from the one to which they were currently attached. This suggests that FWEs are being transferred, especially in urban areas, which again goes against the original idea of the programme.

Although the minimum educational requirement is seven years of schooling, in 1987 nearly 40 per cent of FWEs had a higher qualification. This change probably reflects the expansion of education opportunities in Botswana in the 1970s and 1980s. However, it also raises a question about job satisfaction. Kenyon (1986), for example, suggests that FWEs with higher than standard seven qualifications may feel restless and less satisfied with their role after a few years. This may be reflected in the increasing requests for transfers.

In summary, about half the existing FWEs have been selected either by health staff applying for the job themselves or through promotion, rather than being selected by their own communities. Over a third of FWEs have more than the minimum educational requirements. The existence of transfers on a fairly large scale, combined with actual selection practice, confirms the general impression that FWEs have tended to become primarily civil servants rather than community representatives.

Basic training

FWEs are trained at Sebele, a rural training centre for extension workers, some 20 km from Gaborone. Between 1971 and 1986 the course was a twelve-week one, including three weeks' fieldwork, usually in a large village health centre. In 1987 the course was increased to sixteen weeks, including four weeks' fieldwork. While in training, FWEs receive a small per diem from Unicef and their local sponsoring council; the council also pays their travel costs. A few FWEs are sponsored by the MOH or other organizations, such as the Botswana Defence Force.

Terms of pay and conditions

Ninety-six per cent of FWEs work either in a health post or a clinic, where they are employed by the district or town council. As we have seen, they therefore fall under the auspices of the ULGS. The remaining FWEs work either in health centres or hospitals, where they are employed by the MOH. Whichever ministry employs them, however, FWEs are permanent and pensionable civil servants on a government salary which increases incrementally. The main theoretical difference between FWEs and other 'permanent and pensionable' civil servants is that they should not be transferred out of their community, but we have already noted that this rule is not strictly adhered to.

Given their low minimum educational requirements at entry, and their short training, FWEs are on a relatively high salary scale compared with other civil servants. In 1987 a senior FWE on maximum salary earned 6,852 pula (1713 US $) per annum, whereas a junior enrolled nurse on minimum salary earned 3,408 pula (852 US $). This appears to have come about following pressure from the early proponents of the programme at the start of the 1970s, and possibly in response to the demand for FWEs from district councils. It has sometimes led to controversy between FWEs and some of their enrolled nurse supervisors, as occasionally a senior FWE may be earning more than her supervisor.

Family welfare educator activities

Facility-based activities
Although activities vary between health facilities, FWEs mainly participate in the registration of patients, weighing, taking blood pressure, administering dressings and sometimes dispensing drugs. They are also involved in record-keeping for the facility. When working on their own in a health post, they conduct patient consultations and may prescribe from a limited range of drugs. However, their major role within the facilities is generally seen as the running of child welfare clinics. Some community members see these clinics as the FWEs' only task, and some nurses leave child welfare activities within their facility (except immunization) completely to the FWEs. FWEs have expressed a strong preference for this type of care although they, some nurses and some community members also mentioned FWE health talks, health education and direct feeding (distribution of free food during periods of drought) as being both enjoyable and productive activities.

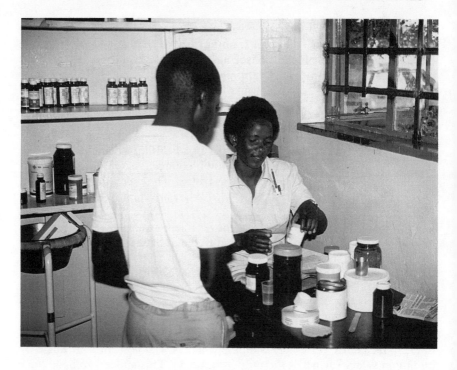

7 *A familiar role for family welfare educators is dispensing drugs in the health facility. Photo: David Ross (London School of Hygiene).*

Home visiting

There was some conflict in the evidence on the numbers of home visits undertaken by FWEs: FWE responses to the self-administered questionnaire and the examination of home-visit records did not always tally. Of 514 FWEs who answered this question, 56 per cent reported doing less than five visits in the previous week, 29 per cent did between five and nine visits, and only 15 per cent reported doing 10 or more visits. The mean number of visits reported was 5.4, which would be equivalent to 21.6 per month. This figure was higher than that obtained from examination of twenty-five FWEs' record books, from which the mean monthly number of visits was estimated to be 8.8.

The number of home visits per week reported by FWEs varied according to the type of facility in which they were based. Perhaps surprisingly, it was highest when they worked in a health post without an enrolled nurse and lowest when they worked in a health centre or hospital. Indeed, more home visits per week were undertaken when they worked in a health post without an enrolled nurse than when they worked alongside one. It is difficult to interpret the meaning of these findings: perhaps loneliness drives the FWE to visit community members in their homes, while the company of an enrolled nurse increases the potential for offering treatment at the health post. In theory, of course, the presence of other health workers should free FWEs to make home visits.

Nearly three-quarters of the home visits made with the researcher in this study were in the morning; this was the time the FWEs preferred as it was cooler. The majority of these visits lasted thirty minutes or less, with none lasting longer than one hour.

What do FWEs do on such visits? Interestingly, the great majority are initiated from the base health facility. This study found that 50 per cent of visits were undertaken to trace defaulters from tuberculosis, psychiatric, antenatal, child welfare or direct-feeding programmes, and 34 per cent to provide continuing care for patients who had previously attended the facility or who were previously known to need care, such as the elderly or disabled. A further 9 per cent of visits were in connection with a survey of household sanitation facilities which had been taking place during the survey period in the area. This bias towards home visits being initiated from the health facility rather than being undertaken on a routine basis is not a recent phenomenon. As early as 1973, an evaluation noted 'that FWEs spend a greater proportion of their time on home visiting for follow up of family planning clients, tuberculosis contacts etc' (Cook 1973).

None of the twenty-five FWEs interviewed had an established system by which they made routine home visits. Only one of them was able to produce a map showing all the households for which she was responsible, and most FWEs were unable to estimate the approximate number of households in their area. These findings probably underline some feeling of ambivalence on the part of FWEs as to their right to visit households as a matter of routine, rather than just to follow up a known problem. They certainly raise questions about the value of home visits. For example, it was clear that the attitudes and manner of the FWEs were likely to have an important effect on the quality of communication which occurred during the visit; a wide variation in the standard of communication was observed.

While some FWEs are sympathetic, providing encouragement and practical advice, others may be aggressive and put forward little or no explanation for their advice. Even on a first visit to a household, some failed to introduce themselves or to make their reason for visiting clear. Often it seemed that a mental checklist of standard activities to be undertaken during a home visit was used by the FWE, irrespective of whether all of it was relevant to the particular situation. Negative reactions from households to such visits were expressed in group discussions with community members. Some saw visits as rude and intrusive.

Who does the FWE visit? Only 20 per cent of the households interviewed where a home visit could be confirmed to have taken place during the previous month included a relative of the FWE. None of these, moreover, was closer than the FWE's uncle or first cousin, and most were distant cousins. FWEs do not appear, therefore, to favour their own family when undertaking home visits. Indeed, FWEs expressed their difficulty in confronting their own families, particularly on delicate issues such as family

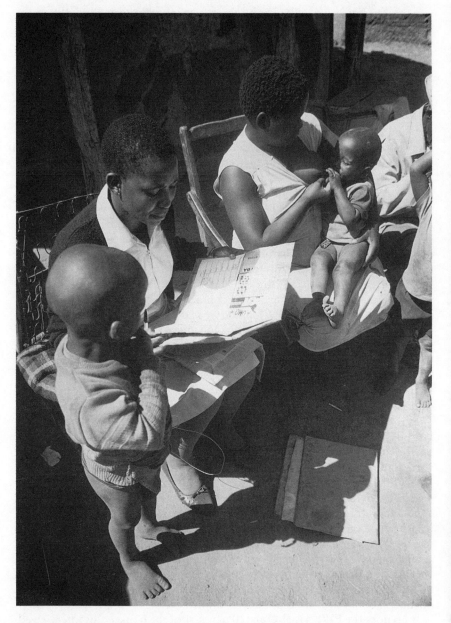

8   *In a follow-up visit to a household, the family welfare educator records the family's immunization status. Photo: Lucy Gilson (London School of Hygiene).*

planning and sexually transmitted diseases. On the other hand, it was not clear whether the families that were visited were those most in need of support.

So how do FWEs divide their time between home visits and facilities? In the national questionnaire, the answers were fairly evenly divided: 51 per cent said they spent more time home visiting, and 49 per cent said working in the facility was their main occupation. As the questionnaire was self-administered this result is probably not a true reflection of actual activities: it is more likely to reflect FWEs' expectations of what they 'should' answer.

As we have already seen, actual observations during this and previous studies (such as Bennett *et al.* 1980; Manyeneng 1982; Owuor-Omondi *et al.* 1986) indicate that the FWEs are spending the great majority of their time in the health facilities. Ninety-one per cent of the home visits recorded were estimated to be within 2 km of the health facility. Walking time to home visits seldom exceeded thirty minutes. It is probably realistic to say that the average FWE spends less than 10 per cent of her time undertaking home visits, including travelling time to and from the households.

Other community-based activities
If FWEs spend a limited amount of time visiting households, do they nevertheless have contact with the local institutions in the village, such as the village development or health committees? Again, links seem tenuous. According to the national questionnaire, almost half the FWEs had not met with the VDC, and almost a third had not met with the VHC within the last three months. This limited contact between these village committees and the FWEs was confirmed in interviews with members of the committees. It cannot entirely be laid at the door of the FWEs, but partly reflects the widespread inactivity of these committees. Only 34 per cent of the FWEs reported that the VHC in their community was active. Owuor-Omondi *et al.* (1987) found that only 37 per cent of the VHC members interviewed reported that their VHC was active and had a clear plan of activities. It is difficult to know whether VHCs would be more active if FWEs were to have more frequent meetings with them, or whether FWEs do not meet with them because they proved inactive in the past.

Although contacts with the VHCs are low, the great majority of FWEs say that they belong to at least one community organization excluding the VHC or VDC. They do, therefore, have contact with community groups outside their working hours.

Family welfare educators' activity preferences

When asked with which activity they preferred to be involved, 90 per cent of FWEs came down in favour of home visiting. This was in agreement with earlier findings. Again, it is difficult to decide to what extent these reported preferences may have been influenced by the FWEs' perceptions of what they felt they 'should' answer to this question. Although no clear answer to the problem emerged from focus-group discussions with FWEs, there were hints that their stated preference for home visiting may well have been biased for this reason. In at least one discussion, the home-visiting preference was challenged by one FWE who suggested to her colleagues that this was not true; several FWEs then admitted that they did not like home visiting because it necessitated walking around the village, often in hot and sandy conditions. The discrepancy between stated preferences and the reality of the low number of home visits raises questions about the extent to which FWEs genuinely prefer visiting households.

Community perceptions

Conflicting further with the FWEs' stated preference for home visiting, community members overwhelmingly considered their facility-based work to be their main and most important role. This was the unequivocal finding of questionnaires sent to VDC, VHC and other community members. Although home visiting was not seen as unimportant, community members felt that it was of secondary importance only. In those villages where FWEs worked in a health post without an enrolled nurse, community members felt strongly that she should remain there throughout normal working hours in case a sick person needed her attention.

Support and supervision

As we saw in Chapter 3, support and supervision of CHWs are considered to be the most essential components in making a programme effective. In Botswana, the FWEs working in clinics and health posts with an enrolled nurse receive day-to-day supervision from the local nurses with whom they are working. Most of this supervision relates to the FWEs' facility-based activities, as many enrolled nurses have no training or experience of community-based work and are therefore ill placed to supervise these aspects of FWEs' work. Furthermore, as we have seen, most nurses tend to encourage FWEs to spend time in the health facilities to assist them with their duties. FWEs who work in a health post without an enrolled nurse do not receive any day-to-day supervision, although sometimes they are visited by nurses from neighbouring clinics.

All FWEs receive occasional supervisory visits from a wide variety of district- and regional-level staff, including district council matrons, senior nursing sisters, CHNs and other members of the regional health team. Lines of accountability are unclear, however, and this has been exacerbated by uncertainties over the role and status of the CHNs on the regional health teams in relation to other senior nursing cadres (Anderson 1986). In general, the FWEs tend to consider the nurses with whom they work on a daily basis – or those from the nearest clinic – to be their main supervisors.

Needless to say, quality of supervision is variable. It is rare for FWEs to be supervised on home visits or other community-based activities, apart perhaps from having their home-visiting record books checked. This confirms the previous findings of Owuor-Omondi et al. (1986) that only

17.5 per cent of the FWEs they interviewed were satisfied with the supervision they received, and that the commonest suggestion as to how this supervision could be made more beneficial was that the supervisor should accompany them on home visits, or be present when they addressed community meetings or VHCs. The inadequacy of support for such activities partly reflects the attitudes of supervisors. Even among the CHNs on the regional health teams – who should be the most community-orientated of all nurses – only two out of seventeen who responded to a questionnaire put a community-based activity at the top of a list of the FWEs' most important tasks.

Other constraints on supervision lie with a lack of vehicles to make journeys to remote health posts. Some clinics have avoided this problem by holding regular monthly or two-monthly meetings at the clinic, attended by all the FWEs from the catchment area. Unfortunately, this is by no means a universal practice, and even when such meetings do occur they may be dominated by administrative matters rather than used for the discussion of FWEs' problems or for in-service training.

In 1987 and 1988 efforts were being made to improve the support and supervision of FWEs. Country-wide workshops, funded by the World Bank, were held for both council and regional health team staff in order to clarify the FWEs' main roles. The organizers of these workshops hope that all the FWEs' potential supervisors will have received some reorientation on how they might support and supervise the FWEs better. It remains to be seen how much impact this will have on the actual practices of the supervisors and on the FWEs themselves.

In-service training

The in-service training or continuing education of FWEs is co-ordinated by the CHNs from the regional health teams. This has mainly been limited to one- or two-day seminars conducted every few months. Few FWEs have ever received a refresher course or retraining to give them the skills to perform tasks which have been added to their responsibilities since they received their basic training. However, some refresher and reorientation courses were included in the World Bank programme discussed above.

Costs of family welfare educators and their activities

Given their integrated role within health facilities it is both difficult and inappropriate to cost FWEs separately from the facilities. It is clear, however, that of the costs attached to the FWEs alone the dominant input cost is for salaries, and the other main cost is for basic training. FWEs use no supplies outside their base facility, receive no supervision of their home visiting and have little in-service training.

To get a better idea of the total costs associated with FWEs' activities, a sample of facilities in one district was examined. This included two clinics, two health posts with enrolled nurses and one health post with only an FWE.

It is clear that recurrent expenditures are the major annual costs for all facilities (83–95 per cent), and that salaries are the dominant input cost in most facilities (65–78 per cent). In all but one of the facilities, FWE salaries alone represented over 20 per cent of total costs, emphasizing the importance of FWEs as an available resource within the facility. For all facilities, drugs were the second most important item of expenditure – although ranging from 8 to 31 per cent of total costs. Supervision costs (based on an average of two half-day visits per month) were also estimated to be a significant portion of the total costs of facilities where FWEs work alone (around 15 per cent). The main influence over this cost in all facilities would be their distance from the supervisor's base.

Conclusions

It is clear that FWEs have moved a long way from how they were originally envisaged – as health workers in the community, with half their time spent in facilities. The big question being asked in Botswana, therefore, is how feasible is it to make FWEs more community-orientated? Let us consider three ways of answering this question: 1 by considering the opinions of a range of health workers and community members; 2 by an analysis of the outpatient workload of selected facilities; and 3 by an assessment of the efficiency of resource use within facilities.

Health workers' and community members' views

As one might predict, there was almost unanimous approval from policy-makers and health workers for the suggestion that the FWEs should do more home-visiting and other community-based activities, and spend less time working in the health facilities. At the same time, however, there was strong consensus that the FWEs could only do so if they were replaced in the health facilities, preferably by enrolled nurses. Although this step was felt to be most crucial when FWEs were working in a health post without an enrolled nurse, they were also thought to be playing a vital role when they worked in a health post alongside an enrolled nurse or in a clinic.

There was almost unanimous agreement, both among health workers and community members, that FWEs should continue to have a daily link with their local health facility, and that they should continue to carry out some clinical activities within that facility. How realistic these enthusiams are is very questionable, as such links will probably result in the FWEs' community activities becoming marginalized, as has happened in the 1970s and 1980s. Since they are seen as useful extra pairs of hands in the facilities, there is no reason to believe that they will be released or encouraged to do work in the community. If they were replaced in the facilities there might be more chance of community work replacing facility work, but the cost implications for the MOH are enormous. It has to be remembered that over half of the 45 per cent of FWEs who work in health posts, work alone, and to replace them, as well as those making a contribution within larger health facilities, would be a major undertaking.

Outpatient workload

The nurses expressed great appreciation of the assistance they got from FWEs in their busy clinics. How busy were the nurses and could they do without their FWEs?

Each year, each health facility reports the number of patient contacts (including contacts at mobile clinics carried out by their staff) to the Health Statistics Unit within the MOH. They also report their actual staff in post on 31 December each year. These data for 1986 were studied for fourteen health facilities. They were used to provide objective evidence as to whether or not the facilities were so overloaded as to prohibit the FWEs' being released to carry out more community-based activities, such as home visiting. The outpatient contacts included child welfare, family planning, antenatal and postnatal clinics, as well as contacts by sick patients. In the calculations it was assumed that all outpatient contacts occurred during the five days from Monday to Friday each week (i.e. 260 days per year), and that each nurse or FWE was available for clinical work on all these days (i.e. not allowing any days for staff absences).

Using these assumptions, and the data for 1986, the mean number of outpatient contacts per working day per 'clinical staff member' (i.e. nurses and FWEs), and per nurse (i.e. excluding FWEs), was calculated for each of the fourteen health facilities.

The results showed that, overall, there was relatively little difference between the mean workloads of the different types of facility: clinics 13.2 outpatient visits per clinical staff member per day; health posts with an enrolled nurse, 15.2; and health posts without an enrolled nurse, 17.2. On the other hand, there was considerable variation in the workload per clinical staff member among individual facilities of the same type.

It is difficult to determine what might be a reasonable number of patient contacts per clinical staff member per day, and professionals differ widely in what they think is acceptable. For the sake of argument we took the acceptable range to be between thirty and forty-five patient contacts per clinical staff member per working day. If one assumes that each clinical staff member spends six hours seeing patients per day, allowing the remaining two working hours per day for administration, breaks, and so on, then this range corresponds to a mean of between 5 and 7.5 patients per hour, or one patient contact per 8–12 minutes.

This fairly generous time allocation has been chosen to allow for the variation in the workload which is bound to occur from day to day. Even if twice the acceptable maximum mean number of patients were to come on one day, then this would only amount to ninety patient contacts per clinical staff member, or one contact every four minutes.

During 1986 the mean workload of all the fourteen health facilities fell below thirty patients per day. If one excludes the health posts without an enrolled nurse, where removal of the FWE from all facility-based activities would obviously leave the health post without a clinical staff member, then even if all the FWEs had been released from clinical duties, only one of the health facilities would have exceeded a mean of forty-five patient contacts per nurse per day.

In conclusion, all the fourteen clinics and health posts we examined would appear to be overstaffed, if their sole role is to see outpatients. So the outpatient workload should not be a valid constraint to FWEs' doing more community-based activities, at least within these particular facilities.

Efficiency of resource use

Finally, what impact do current staffing patterns have on costs? If average costs (costs per contact) are examined more closely, the influence of staff costs on operational efficiency (measured by average costs) can be seen. For two health posts with an enrolled nurse and FWE, average costs at one were about two-thirds those of the other. The main cause of this difference was the higher salary cost per contact (3.39 pula (0.9 US $) versus 2.13 pula (0.5 US $)), resulting from the higher utilization of one health post given the same staffing level. Not only does this suggest that one health post was relatively overstaffed for its workload, but also that the resource of personnel, in particular, could be used more efficiently if utilization within all facilities were increased, or if FWEs were to have an enlarged role outside the facilities. Such a role would justify the inclusion of their community-based activities in the assessment of operational efficiency. Moreover, if FWEs were to work more outside the facilities, their activities might well lead to increased use of the facilities and so to improved efficiency of resource use both inside and outside them.

The conclusion seems to be that not only is it feasible for FWEs to do more community-based activities, but that if they did, it could improve the efficiency with which they and other health resources are used, ensuring better value for money. However, in order for FWEs to be effective in this role it would be necessary to improve their support and supervision, ensuring greater frequency of contact with supervisors who have the skills to encourage home visiting. But even with such improvements, the attitudes of FWEs, other health workers, and the community towards their role would still need to be confronted. Unless all those connected with FWEs see community-based activities as their first priority it is likely that they will drift back into the facilities in order to fulfil a useful, but not vital, role.

References

Anderson, S. (1986). 'Fra' among community health nurses: a research report. *Botswana National Health Bulletin*, 2, 3, 351–70.

Bennett, J. *et al.* (1980). *Report on Evaluation of Family Welfare Educator's Programme and Internship in Primary Health Care in Botswana.* Ministry of Health, Gaborone.

Colclough, C. and McCarthy, S. (1980). *The Political Economy of Botswana.* Oxford University Press, Oxford.

Cook, S. (1973). *A Report of an Evaluation of the International Planned Parenthood Federation Programme in Botswana 1969–1973.* IPPF/Government of Botswana.

Egner, B. (1987). *The District Councils and Decentralisation 1978–1986.* Report to SIDA and the Ministry of Local Government and Lands, Gaborone.

Egner, B. and Klausen, A.L. (1980). *Poverty in Botswana.* National Institute of Development and Cultural Research. University College of Botswana, Gaborone.

Gish, O. and Walker, G. (1977). *Mobile Health Services.* Tri-Med Books Ltd, London.

Government of Botswana (1972). *Third National Development Plan.* Government Printers, Gaborone.

Government of Botswana/Unicef (1986). *The Situation of Children and Women in Botswana*, Gaborone.

Griffiths, A. (1986). *Financing of Health Services in Botswana* (draft final report). Ministry of Health, Gaborone.

Kenyon, J. (1986). *Family Welfare Educator: Task Oriented Curriculum and Lesson Plans.* Family Health Division, Ministry of Health, Gaborone.

Kromberg, M. (1986). Personal communication.

Manyeneng, W. (1982). *The Botswana Report of the Interregional Study: Research and Development on Community Health Workers.* Ministry of Health, Gaborone.

Ministry of Health (1984). *Health Statistics Report.* Government Printers, Gaborone.

Owuor-Omondi, L., Atlaholang, D. and Diseko, R. (1986). *The Changing Role of Family Welfare Educators?: An Evaluation of the Role of FWEs in the Implementation of Primary Health Care in Botswana.* National Health Status Evaluation Monograph Series, 1. Ministry of Health, Gaborone.

Owuor-Ormondi, L., Atlaholang, D. and Diseko, R. (1987). *Village Health Committees: Viable Instruments of Community Mobilisation for Primary Health Care?* National Health Status Evaluation Monograph Series, 4. Ministry of Health, Gaborone.

8 | Health promoters in Colombia

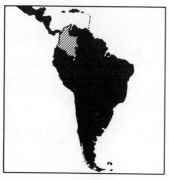

9 Map of South America, with Colombia highlighted. Drawn by Geoff Penna.

Health promoters have existed in Colombia since the 1950s, although the national government programme only began in 1976. They differ from the Botswana community health workers (CHWs) in that nearly all their time is spent visiting people in their homes: only about once a month might they spend a day helping health professionals in a health facility. They work in rural areas and often travel considerable distances to visit families. How effective are they? What is the context within which they work?

Country background

Colombia is located in the extreme northwest of South America and is divided into five distinct regions: the Caribbean coastal plain located to the north; the Pacific coastal plain located to the west; the central Andean region which is predominantly mountainous with long valleys and extensive plains; the Orinoquia region to the east with broad plains and land suitable for cattle raising; and the Amazonian region to the southeast which is predominantly covered by jungle.

Sixty-five per cent of the 28.9 million population now live in urban areas. This proportion is still increasing and has more than doubled within the last fifty years. By the year 2000, it is estimated that at least 75 per cent of the population will be urban. Some of the rural areas are very sparsely populated, especially the Amazonian region.

Socio-economic characteristics

Colombia is a middle-income country: the mean per capita income was estimated at US $1,566 in 1985. Because of the high rates of urbanization, amenities are relatively good: in 1985, 78 per cent of the country's houses were supplied with electricity, 70 per cent with water mains, and 59 per cent with a water-borne sewage disposal system. Needless to say, these figures vary considerably between rural and urban areas, and between the slums and richer areas of the cities.

The literacy rate was estimated at 88 per cent in 1985; 72 per cent of the adult population had completed at least primary education, and 30 per cent secondary school. Full-time employment rates are low, however, particularly for women. In 1984 women represented 42 per cent of the total working force. According to official figures, only 31.6 per cent of the female population of working age are in work (68.3 per cent of the male).

Although Colombia has a substantial international debt, its debt service ratio is not as high as that of several other Latin American countries. The violent crime rate is relatively high, and the number of homicides has increased significantly in recent years. Deaths due to violence are among the top ten causes of mortality in the country as a whole, even when road traffic accidents are excluded.

Health and health services

National health indicators

The rate of growth of the population has declined to 1.9 per cent per year, though 36 per cent of the population were still under fifteen years of age in 1985. The total fertility rate had dropped from 6.7 births per woman at the end of her reproductive age in 1968 to 3.6 in 1980, and it is estimated it will be between 2.0 and 2.5 by the year 2000.

The crude death rate has also dropped substantially from 22.4 per 1000 in 1940 to 9.8 in 1965, and in 1987 was estimated to lie around 5–6 per 1000. According to the Ministry of Health (Ministerio de Salud 1985), the infant mortality rate has fallen from 135 per 1000 in 1950 to 50–55 per 1000 in 1984, and the life expectancy at birth had increased to 63.6 years by 1981.

The maternal mortality rate has dropped from 3.1 per 1000 live births in 1954 to 1.1 per 1000 in 1984, although this rate is still considered unacceptably high. Most births (77 per cent) occurred in official health facilities in 1985. As with many coverage indicators in Colombia, however, the proportion was much lower in rural areas (38 per cent) than in urban. Obstetric conditions make up 40 per cent of all hospital inpatient admissions.

The morbidity pattern of Colombia reflects this recent, rapid transition from a high-fertility, high-mortality country to a relatively low-fertility, low-mortality country, with childhood infectious diseases such as diarrhoea and respiratory tract infections still being common in the poor rural and urban populations, but chronic degenerative diseases – such as heart disease and cancer – assuming increasing importance, especially among the urban middle and upper classes.

According to the national health survey carried out between 1977 and 1980, 40 per cent of all children under five years of age were considered to be malnourished. Most of this was due to stunting (chronic malnutrition), while 6 per cent of all children under five years of age suffered from wasting (acute malnutrition).

Approximately 70 per cent of children between one and two years had received a full course of polio, DPT (Diphtheria, pertussis, tetanus), measles and BCG (tuberculosis) vaccinations in 1984, and 77 per cent of pregnant women were estimated to have received at least two doses of tetanus toxoid. Although the incidence of immunizable diseases in children under one year has varied considerably from year to year, the overall trend has been downward, especially during the 1980s.

The health system

The present national health system was formally set up in 1975, although approximately 16 per cent of the population are also covered by the national employees' social security system, and 9 per cent by other health insurance schemes. Though private practitioners are also utilized by a wide variety of people, only 5 per cent of the population are estimated to rely on them as their major source of health care.

The Colombian health system is divided into national, provincial, regional and local levels. There are some 107 regional hospitals, and at the local level the main health facilities are either a small hospital and/or health centres/health posts. The rural (local-level) health centres, of which there are more than 3,000 in the country, are usually staffed by an auxiliary nurse with eighteen months' training. A medical doctor should visit such a centre once a week. Below this level, though relating to the health centre or local hospital, are the community-based health promoters.

There has been a gradual expansion of the health services in recent decades, and this has been accompanied by an expansion of government health personnel. Interestingly, there are almost four times as many doctors as professional nurses, and almost as many doctors as auxiliary nurses in the country. As a national average there are eight doctors per 10,000 people, but 84 per cent of all doctors are located in the country's five largest cities. In addition to the formal health care personnel, including the health promoters, there are an estimated 6,250 traditional midwives, of whom half have received some official training. Within the 1980s there has been a rapid increase in the services being provided to isolated rural and marginal urban areas. There is a policy by which doctors, nurses and dentists must spend a year providing 'social service' in the rural areas immediately after they qualify, and the rural health services are heavily dependent on these inexperienced professionals.

The primary health care (PHC) facilities (*unidades primarias de atención*, or UPAs) expanded enormously over the period 1976 to 1984, increasing coverage from 1 to 9 million inhabitants in poor rural and urban areas. These UPAs usually consist of a clinic or health centre staffed mainly by auxiliary nurses, to which a number of health promoters are attached. A UPA may also be headed by a local hospital. Children under five years, and women between fifteen and forty-four years, are supposed to receive special attention in terms of the services provided (Ministerio de Salud 1984; 1987).

Historical development of the health promoter (*promotora de salud*) programme

The increasing international interest in peripheral and community-based health care of the past three decades also occurred within Colombia, which formally adopted the PHC strategy under the title *Atención Primaria de Salud*. As in most developing countries, the CHW has been seen as a key health cadre for the extension of health service coverage, especially within dispersed rural populations. The main category of CHWs in Colombia is the full-time *promotora de salud*, or health promoter.

One of the earliest health promoter schemes in Colombia was initiated in 1958 by the University of Antioquia in the environs of Medellín (Ministerio de Salud 1981). The health promoters, who were mainly young women, were selected by the communities and worked without payment after a brief training period.

A number of other local or regional programmes were also set up in different parts of the country from the 1950s onwards. Most of these were small programmes that trained and deployed community members – usually women – to work as CHWs. These programmes were not evenly distributed throughout Colombia, and although some received government support, most were initiated by private organizations or universities. There was considerable variety in the training, job descriptions and activities of CHWs in the different programmes. Although a few attempted to foster community participation, self-reliance and empowerment, the focus of most programmes was on providing preventive health care through health education and immunization campaigns. Depending on the sponsoring agencies' ability to supervise and supply these early CHWs, it was clear that many of them provided a significant service to the small populations within their catchment areas (Bond 1985; Valle del Cauca 1980).

One of the universities that initiated such a programme was the Universidad del Valle. Other programmes were started by non-governmental agencies such as churches or charities. A health promoter programme of special note, still in operation, is the one sponsored by the

Coffee Growers' Association of Quindio province. This association's health education programme is particularly impressive, with sixty health messages being broadcast by radio each day, and a series of manuals for the health promoters as well as flip charts and illustrated books for use in health education sessions.

Based mainly on the experiences in Antioquia, the Ministerio de Salud initiated a national health promoter programme in 1969, with the Ministry's maternal and child health division taking particular responsibility for the programme. Initially the health promoters were full-time unpaid volunteers, and attrition rates were high. Partly because of this, and partly due to their own demands, they became employees of the Ministerio de Salud in 1976, receiving a regular salary equivalent to the local government minimum wage, and a uniform.

After a rapid expansion in the number of health promoters during the 1970s, numbers stabilized at between 5,000 and 5,300 during the 1980s, largely because of financial constraints placed on the Ministerio de Salud. In 1987 there were estimated to be 5,310 health promoters, of whom 4,816 (90.7 per cent) worked in rural communities, covering an average of 2,100 people.

The health promoters' main officially prescribed role has been to carry out preventive medicine, principally through home visiting. A map and current population census of their area are therefore essential aids. Most health promoters work from home, or from a small health post where they are the sole medical personnel. The day is divided between six hours spent home visiting and two hours' administrative duties. Health promoters are usually equipped with a very limited number of drugs and supplies – such as aspirin, anti-helminthics and bandages – but not, for example, with antibiotics. The number of health promoters with even the minimal amount of basic drugs and equipment decreased between 1979 and 1984 (Table 12).

Health promoters are expected to treat simple ailments and refer patients with complications. They keep a record of all cases as well as a community

Table 12 Available working equipment for health promoters, Colombia, 1979 and 1984.

	1979		1984	
	No.	(%)	No.	(%)
HPs with box of drugs and equipment	454	79.9	208[1]	18.6
HPs without box of drugs and equipment	114	20.1	909	81.4
Total	568	100.0	1117	100.0

[1] Includes 8 basic elements, but of 208 only 46 per cent had these in good order.

Source: Ministerio de Salud (1985)

mortality register. All families in their catchment area should be categorized as either high- or low-risk: the frequency with which the health promoter then visits a family depends on their risk category.

New initiatives

In addition to the health promoters, there has been a major drive since the mid-1980s to train large numbers of part-time, volunteer health workers called *vigías de salud* (health scouts) or *voluntarios de salud* (health volunteers). The majority are secondary-school students, and their training is incorporated into the regular school curriculum. They are joined for this work by Red Cross workers, teachers, social workers, priests and even police who receive a very brief training of about one week, which concentrates on six key health messages: immunization; the importance of perinatal care; respiratory disease control; oral rehydration treatment (ORT) for diarrhoea; nutrition, and family planning. The usefulness of these volunteers is not yet known, although a small study in 1987 suggested that the majority did not recognize or make use of opportunities for health education (Pricor 1987).

While this new initiative may warrant further investigation, the health promoters have been in existence for well over twenty years, working mainly in rural areas. Previous evaluations relied on large-scale questionnaire surveys, in which most of the questions were closed (Durana 1985; Ministerio de Salud 1984). The attempt of this study was to look at the promoters in more depth, using a more qualitative approach to explore their role and assess their success. We should first explain the methodology used for the study.

Study methodology

The focus of this study was twofold. The first was to develop and test a selection of methodologies aimed at evaluating the health promoter programme, and the second was to assess the performance of the programme itself so as to provide suggestions for improvements. The study focused on such areas as the selection, training, tasks, supervision and cost of the health promoters, and the acceptability and replicability of the study methodology.

Several qualitative and quantitative methodologies were used at national and provincial level, as well as in-depth studies in two health regions – one in the province of Valle del Cauca (Zarzal region), and one in the province of Cundinamarca (Facatativa region). While these two regions are not fully representative of the whole of a country as diverse as Colombia, the in-depth studies were used to complement the less-detailed national level study. A series of policy interviews was conducted at national level and in selected provinces, and a questionnaire was sent to all the thirty-three directors of the provincial health services. Twenty-four of them responded, and these twenty-four provinces contained 90 per cent of the health promoters in the country. Interviews, questionnaires, and focus-group discussions were conducted with health personnel – including health promoters – at different levels of the health services in the two selected provinces.

Self-administered questionnaires were also sent to certain health officials in each of the thirty-three provinces – provincial medical officers and provincial nursing officers; and doctors and/or nurses directly in charge of the provincial health promoter programme. Structured interviews were conducted in Cundinamarca and Valle del Cauca with the provincial medical officer; the doctor and nurse in charge of the provincial maternal and child health programme; and the training co-ordinator. At the regional level, structured interviews were conducted with the regional medical officer and regional nursing officer, and focus-group discussions were held with supervisors of the health promoters. At the local level, structured interviews were conducted with eight doctors in charge of the local health services; self-administered questionnaires were sent to fifty-six health promoters; and focus-group discussions were held with health promoters. In each province, four communities and their health promoters were selected for particular in-depth study. This involved the researcher staying in the community, interviewing key informants; observing participants; conducting household interviews and focus-group discussions; and making inventories.

The community-based studies were carried out by two public health nurses who were engaged in a masters degree programme in public health at CIMDER, University del Valle, the collaborating institution. An anthropologist also carried out some of the work in Zarzal region.

Health promoter profile

There were 5,310 health promoters in Colombia in 1987, of whom only 494 (9.3 per cent) worked in urban settings. Over 90 per cent were female and the drop-out rate during 1986 had been less than 5 per cent: only 205 health promoters resigned or left their posts.

The profile derived from detailed studies from Facatativa and Zarzal regions – which together had fifty-six health promoters – is illustrated in Table 13.

Selection and qualifications

It became clear during the study that although there were great variations between different parts of the country in the methods of selection of health promoters, there had been very little community involvement in their

Table 13 Profile of health promoters from Facatativa and Zarzal regions, Colombia.

- 76.8% were between 25 and 39 years old
- 60.7% were unmarried
- 66.1% had given birth to at least one child
- 53.5% had completed more than five years' formal education (the minimum requirement)
- 16.0% did not live in the community in which they worked as the health promoter
- 96.4% of the remaining health promoters had lived in their community for at least five years

selection. Where the community had been consulted, it was usually the community action committee which had suggested potential candidates who were then interviewed and set a written examination by the staff of the local or regional hospital. Several health workers claimed that the community action committee frequently selected candidates either for political or kinship reasons rather than on merit. Most agreed, however, that if the community were really going to be involved in the process of selecting their health promoter, health staff would have to explain the health promoter's job more accurately.

Basic training

Health promoters have to be at least eighteen years old and to have completed at least five years' schooling. Training consists of three to four months spent in the auxiliary nurse training school of either the provincial, regional or local hospital. In the country as a whole, training of health promoters takes place at the provincial level in twenty-nine provinces, at regional level in three, and at local hospital level in one.

Both the health promoters and their supervisors agreed that this initial training course was too short and that the content was not always appropriate. A review of the standard curriculum revealed a possible excess of anatomy and physiology and of theoretical teaching in general; practical work was often given little emphasis, and curative skills tended to be favoured over preventive ones. As we have seen, health promoters are expected to spend the majority of their time making home visits and giving health education, and with their minimal medical supplies they can only treat a handful of simple conditions.

Although there are notable exceptions, many training schools follow a standard curriculum irrespective of its relevance to local conditions. This is compounded by the fact that some of the trainers have little practical knowledge of the conditions under which the health promoters will later work, the local pattern of disease, or local concepts of health and illness. Hence they may be unaware of the inappropriateness of some of the training that they give, and certainly, several health promoters felt that they had not been well equipped for their roles as health educators.

In addition, it was felt that the initial training course should be reinforced and extended by a carefully planned system of in-service training. Such courses have been carried out in many regions, but they vary substantially in frequency and content. In Zarzal region, for example, nine out of thirty-one health promoters who were interviewed had never attended a course, and only five had attended more than two courses since they started work, whereas in Facatativa region all twenty-two health promoters had been to at least one course, and twenty of them had attended more than two courses.

But yet again, some of those responsible for organizing the in-service training for health promoters had insufficient knowledge of their needs and did not put a great deal of thought into what these might be. In many areas, in-service training courses were not routinely planned or budgeted and were only organized on an *ad hoc* basis if funds became available.

Terms of pay and promotion possibilities

Health promoters wear uniforms and are salaried members of the Ministerio de Salud, with pension and accompanying rights. Although not very high, the salary is attractive to many rural women for whom employment opportunities are few, and this is reflected in the low attrition rates among health promoters. However, they do not receive any annual increments and have no prospects for promotion, for example, to auxiliary nurse, without further training. They are given no concessions should they apply for auxiliary nurse training, however, and must attend the entire two-year course.

Health promoter activities

Home visiting
We have seen that most health promoters spend the majority of their time making home visits. However, the average number of visits per day was only four in the rural-area studies. Although the content of visits varies considerably, promoters usually review the general health of the household members, paying special attention to the women and children. They check immunization status, and attendance at child, antenatal or postnatal clinics. General hygiene and sanitation standards may be reviewed and discussed, and the health promoter may give a short teaching session on a topic such as prevention and treatment of diarrhoea, or family planning, though they rarely have any visual aids or other educational materials to help them. None of the health promoters in the two areas we studied carried weighing scales on their visits, and although some had arm-circumference tapes (for assessing body-fat) they did not use these routinely. The great majority of community members seemed to value these home visits and the work of the health promoters in general, though they would have preferred it if the health promoters had a greater curative capacity than their small first-aid kits allowed.

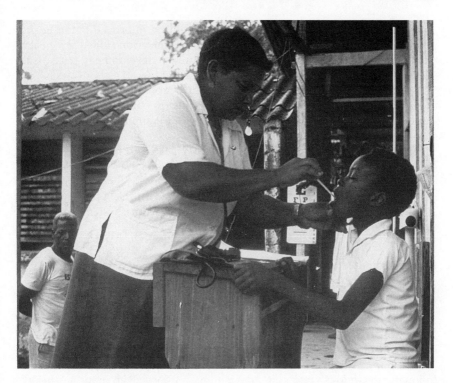

10 Health promoters in Colombia spend considerable time treating people in the households they visit. Here a boy has his temperature taken. Photo: P.E.M. Engelkes (Royal Tropical Institute, Amsterdam).

Home visits are not cheap, especially in dispersed rural communities where walking times to the households are substantial. A detailed study of health service recurrent costs in 1986 in the province of Valle del Cauca (Zarzal region) showed that each rural home visit cost an average of 395 pesos (US $1.80), and each urban visit cost an average of 191 pesos (US $0.87) (Salazar et al. 1987). Although the types of contact are not the same, of course, it is interesting to note that the same study found that the average recurrent cost to the health services of a consultation with a doctor was 203 pesos (US $0.92), with a nurse 131 pesos (US $0.60), and with a dentist 280 pesos (US $1.27), while the average cost of a vaccination for a child was 252 pesos (US $1.15) (Salazar et al. 1987). This study was based on a detailed time and motion study of all categories of health staff, and proportional allocation of all recurrent costs to the health services of each activity. It did not, however, include the costs incurred by the community members concerned.

Other community-based activities
Most health promoters also give occasional health talks to members of the

community. The varied attendance rates could be improved if the health promoters were given specific training in communication skills. Few health promoters were involved in general community development tasks, and most confined their work to health-related activities.

Contrary to their job description, many promoters are increasingly spending a substantial proportion of their time on curative activities, even during home visits, although lack of drugs and equipment clearly restrict this.

We saw above that health promoters are expected to refer patients with complications to the nearest health centre or hospital. Many of them complained that their patients were not given any preferential treatment over those who had attended of their own accord. Where preferential treatment was given, as in Facatativa region, the referral system functioned much better.

Health promoter activity preference and community perceptions

Health promoters perceived the following to be their most important tasks: home visiting; health education; checking immunization; promotion of the use of the health services; and general maternal and child health activities. Their preferred activities were checking vaccinations; maternal and child-health consultations; health education; and home visiting (Table 14).

Community members indicated that the health promoters performed the following activities best (in descending order): vaccination; health education; home visiting; and maternal and child health. We have already seen, however, that many health promoters would like to have access to additional drugs and further training to be able to perform more curative tasks, and that this would also be valued by the communities with which they work.

Support and supervision

The area in which the most problems were identified – both by the health promoters and by others – was in their support and supervision. This is despite the fact that most health promoters have reasonably frequent contact with supervisory staff. Among the fifty-six health promoters interviewed in detail in Zarzal and Facatativa Regions, for example, 86 per cent had received at least one visit from a nurse or auxiliary nurse within the last three months, and 66 per cent had received at least three visits. The majority (74 per cent) of these visits lasted at least three hours. In addition, a number of villages where health promoters worked were visited on a regular basis by a team from the local hospital or health centre, but when this happened the promoters tended to be involved mainly in administrative tasks to assist the doctor or nurse.

Most of the supervisory visits to the health promoters were made by auxiliary nurses, although in some areas this role was performed by the

Table 14 Health promoters' most important activities, Zarzal and Facatativa regions, Colombia.

Activities	Zarzal		Facatativa		Total	
	No.	(%)	No.	(%)	No.	(%)
General						
home visiting	27	81.8	12	52.2	39	69.6
making a census	–	–	18	78.3	18	32.1
Curative care						
injections	16	48.5	4	17.4	20	35.7
curative care	16	48.5	–	–	16	28.6
refer patients	–	–	15	65.2	15	26.8
give treatment	–	–	5	21.7	5	8.9
first aid	7	21.2	2	8.7	9	16.1
assisting in child delivery	3	9.1	–	–	3	5.4
Prevention and promotion						
health education	23	69.7	15	65.2	38	67.9
immunization	29	87.9	3	13.0	32	57.1
promotion of health services	14	42.4	14	60.9	28	50.0
MCH activities	15	45.5	10	43.5	25	44.6
work with the community	5	15.2	–	–	5	8.9
patient follow-up	3	9.1	–	–	3	5.4
knowing the community	3	9.1	–	–	3	5.4
Administrative work activity						
planning	–	–	1	4.3	1	1.8
Total informants	33		23		56	

nurse doing her social service year. Few of the auxiliary nurses had received much training in supervision, and even fewer in how to give support to the health promoters. Supervisory visits tended to emphasize checking records and taking an inventory of the health promoter's equipment. Although the supervisor sometimes gave a short, pre-prepared educational talk, and asked whether the health promoter had any problems, these were usually dealt with in a fairly cursory manner and, anyway, the supervisor often did not have the ability to solve the problems. It was rare for a supervisor to accompany the health promoter on a home visit, or to hold a community meeting with her. Thus, with notable local exceptions, the supervision – like the initial training of the health promoter – tended to be theoretical, didactic and critical, rather than practical and supportive.

Responses from the health promoters indicated that at least half of them did not feel particularly valued by other health personnel. The following statements were indicative: 'We are accepted but not valued'; 'They do not realize what we do'; 'Senior doctors and nurses never come to the village to see with their own eyes what we actually do'.

As well as the supervisory visits they receive at their health posts, however, the great majority of health promoters attend regular monthly meetings with their supervisors and other health promoters in their local health centre or hospital. These monthly meetings are often under the direct control of the nurse doing her social service year. Since she has just qualified, and has usually had no previous experience of working in a rural area, she is generally very poorly equipped for the role. She often resorts to the didactic teaching of subjects she herself has recently been taught, many of which are again either inappropriate or irrelevant to the health promoter. The remainder of the monthly meeting is usually taken up with the payment of salaries, checking records, forms and monthly reports, planning the next month's activities, and other administrative tasks – such as the supplying of uniforms. Since nurses doing their social service year rarely stay in a rural area for longer than a year there is a serious lack of continuity in the supervision and informal in-service training of health promoters. In summary, the main problems with the supervision of the health promoters have less to do with the number of contacts with the supervisor than with the quality of these contacts.

The health promoters also receive varying levels of support from their local community and its institutions. This is most commonly of a passive nature, such as attending the health promoter's talks or vaccination sessions. In general, the community sees the health promoter as a member of the government health services. Yet the health services sometimes claim that they cannot easily sanction or sack an incompetent health promoter because of the probable political consequences – as he or she is likely to be related to important local families. This problem of patronage, however, is by no means confined to health promoters within the government services.

It is not only supervision that fails the health promoters' needs. Their supplies (and even their salaries) are often delayed or inadequate. This is a widespread problem for all the peripheral health services, especially in the poorer regions of the country. In the major city hospitals, failure to pay salaries has immediate political repercussions, as does a lack of equipment or supplies. Rural communities are more distant and therefore easier to ignore. A recent study in Zarzal region showed that 89.4 per cent of the recurrent expenditure of the *unidad local* of Toro in 1985 (peripheral health services for a population of 13,589 based on a local hospital) had been spent on staff salaries and benefits, 8.1 per cent on expenses and allowances, and only 2.5 per cent on drugs and supplies (Salazar *et al.* 1987). Since the health promoter is at the end of the long chain of supply, he or she is usually the first to suffer when supplies are inadequate. Several of the health promoters we visited did not have key items of equipment such as a thermometer, gauze and dressing plasters, and more than half of this small sample did not have packets of oral rehydration salts.

In-service training

As discussed above, in-service training leaves much to be desired. Courses have been held in many regions, but they vary in frequency and content.

According to Ministerio de Salud sources, between 1985 and 1987 forty-four in-service training courses were provided for health promoters in twenty-eight of the thirty-three provinces. The courses focused on such topics as 'Family planning', 'Use of the health scout's manual' (*manual del vigía*)', 'The national plan for child survival' and 'Maternal and child health'. These courses had been given sporadically, however, and often with insufficient planning. Little attention was given to providing in-service training courses that related directly to specific problems faced by health promoters in a particular area.

Record-keeping and the information system

The health promoters themselves, as well as their supervisors and the health managers, indicated that the present system of record-keeping and information-gathering needed to be reviewed and revised. All felt that the health promoters had to complete too many different forms and to gather too much information. Some health promoters are required to complete as many as eighteen different forms each month. A great deal of this information is not used either by the health promoters in evaluating and planning their own work, or by other health service staff. Valuable time spent filling out forms could be significantly reduced by consolidating record-keeping and by improving the health promoters' information-gathering techniques. Helpful responses from supervisors who have received such records would greatly assist the health promoters, indicating to them the kinds of information that are important.

Should the health promoters' job description be re-evaluated?

Even though most communities' acceptance of the health promoters was found to be high, many people felt that their activities and capabilities were too limited. Other health personnel also generally accepted the health promoters but did not necessarily value them very highly. The health promoters themselves not only considered that they were often called upon to perform tasks for which they were untrained, but also that they would like to be able to carry out a greater variety of activities than those which they were currently allowed and equipped to do. All this indicates a need to review the health promoter's job description.

In isolated communities, in particular, which is where most health promoters work, there is a desire for more sophisticated curative care, as well as for midwifery services. This is beyond the current training and scope of health promoters. Given the difficulties of transport and referral from such communities, and the communities' expectations, health promoters often feel compelled to take on tasks that are beyond their job description.

Before considering whether a greater number of curative activities should be included in the health promoter's job description, however, it is important to review the quality of the health promoters' performance of

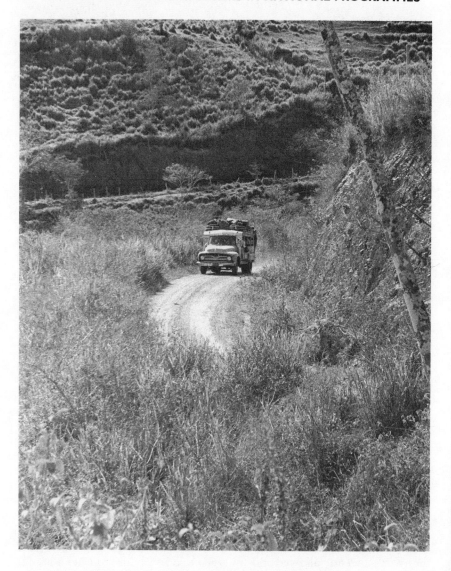

11   *The health promoter is often the only source of medical help close at hand. If members of a household need to visit a health facility they are dependent on getting a lift in a passing vehicle. Photo: David Ross (London School of Hygiene).*

their current activities. Engelkes's (1989) evaluation of promoters in Choco province found that quality of care was low because of lack of support, drugs and equipment, and that there was an underutilization of promoters' services even though over a five-year period their levels of knowledge had improved. In our study we found that health promoters were able to identify the major signs of dehydration, as well as the various factors that could categorize a pregnant woman as belonging in a high-risk group. This supports the suggestion that their knowledge levels are reasonable.

Conclusions

This evaluation showed that, although there is much to commend the health promoter programme in Colombia, there are major problems to be overcome, and changes to be made.

On the one hand, it is certainly true that health promoters have facilitated the extension of basic health services to many of the more remote communities of Colombia which would otherwise have remained unserved by government health services. Despite their limited skills, and the meagre resources at their disposal, the health promoters' work was obviously appreciated by most of the families and community leaders interviewed. The fact that the health promoters originated from within the community meant that they usually remained in their post for several years, giving an important element of continuity to the health services of the rural communities. This is particularly important since many of the other health workers change annually. Furthermore, it is unlikely that other health workers would be willing to be posted long-term to such isolated areas. Most of the health promoters encountered were hard-working, conscientious and dedicated, and their commitment and contribution was the more remarkable precisely because of the various inadequacies and problems noted above: these included the need for improved supervision, support, general management and better incorporation of the health promoters into the overall PHC policy and system of the country.

On the other hand, hard questions have to be asked about the quality and costs of the service given by the health promoters. For example, one of the biggest debates about their value centres on the issue of the balance between their curative and preventive tasks, and where such tasks should be carried out – in the health post or within the home.

Currently most Colombian health promoters spend the majority of their time carrying out home visits, during which their main task is to give general health education, to promote improved hygiene and sanitation within the household, and to promote the use of health services, especially the child health, antenatal, delivery and postnatal clinics. They also carry a small number of largely palliative drugs on their home visits, such as aspirins and cough remedies (when these are in stock).

There is a strong demand from both health promoters and their communities for the promoters to be able to provide more curative care, especially in remote dispersed communities. Provision of antibiotics, and training in delivery care, for example, were a frequent demand. Obviously the health promoters would need to receive further training if they were to have this expanded curative role. To be able to provide curative care when routine home visits are the main contact with the community would be very inefficient, however, since the people who are ill on any one day will not necessarily be in the households to be visited on that particular day. An increase in the curative role of the health promoters is likely, therefore, to lead to their spending more time in the health facilities rather than in making home visits.

A crucial question is what can usefully be included in a home visit, and whether this is likely to provide value for money. For the home visit to be productive, the health promoters will need to be given much more specific instructions and teaching skills than they have at present. These would need periodic updating and changing if they were not to become repetitive and boring – both for the promoter and the household. They would also have to be locally acceptable and realistic. For example, since it is unreasonable to expect a person who struggles to feed and clothe his or her family to contemplate buying the materials needed for the construction of a latrine, so the health promoters would need to be given skills to tailor their messages to the reality of the family they are visiting. As well as promoting the use of the formal health services, it would be important to stress and encourage self-reliance. The health promoters could help the community members improve the basic care which they can give to one of their own family who may be ill. This could include simple remedies for diarrhoea, fever, cough, injuries and so on, and an improved knowledge of the early symptoms that should prompt the seeking of care outside the home.

Recent studies have shown that simple diagnostic procedures, based on the history of the illness or on observations that do not require any equipment, can be very effective predictors of, for example, both diarrhoea episodes needing antibiotic treatment (Ronsmans et al. 1988) and pneumonia, at least in young children (Cherian et al. 1988).

Whether or not the provision of preventive and promotive activities by the health promoters will be sufficient will depend to a large degree on the quality and accessibility of other sources of clinical care, such as clinics, health centres and hospitals. This will not only depend on distance, but also on their cultural acceptability, and the social and financial costs to the users. In general, the more accessible these facilities are, the less health promoters will need to provide clinical services either during home visits or from their health posts. However, it is often the very families for whom these health facilities are inaccessible, such as the poorest or most distant, who could benefit from the health promoters' preventive and promotive home visits as well as curative care. A further problem is that home visiting is relatively expensive, particularly in the more dispersed rural settlements.

Ultimately the decision as to whether or not largely preventive and promotive home visits by the health promoters are enough will have to be based on a balanced assessment of the accessibility of other sources of clinical care, and of the acceptability and costs of providing the health promoters with wider clinical skills and the drugs and supplies that they would need to put these skills into practice.

References

Bond, S.L. (1985). Función de las promotoras de salud en el departmento del Valle de Cauca. *Boletín OPS*, Colombia.

Cherian, R. *et al.* (1988). Evaluation of simple clinical signs for the diagnosis of acute lower respiratory tract infections. *The Lancet* (II), 1–8.

Durana, I. (ed.) (1985). *Encuentro nacional de promotoras de salud.* Fusagasuga. Ministry of Health, Bogotá.

Engelkes, P.E.M. (1989). *Health for All? Evaluation and Monitoring in a Comprehensive Primary Health Care Project in Colombia.* Royal Tropical Institute, Amsterdam.

Ministerio de Salud (1981). *Desarrollo de una política de salud 1971–1981. Informe al honorable congreso de la república.* Ministerio de Salud, Bogotá.

Ministerio de Salud (1984). *Diagnostico de salud: políticas y estretegias.* Ministerio de Salud, Bogotá.

Ministerio de Salud (1985). *Evaluación de extensión de cobertura con servicios de salud 1979–1984.* Ministerio de Salud, Bogotá.

Ministerio de Salud (1987). *Programa materno infantil: hechos y proyecciones.* Ministerio de Salud, Bogotá.

Pricor (1987). *Home visit observations – key to assessing the performance of volunteer health promoters.* Pricor, 1, 1.

Ronsmans, C., Bennish, M.L. and Wierzba, R. (1988). Diagnosis and management of dysentery by community health workers. *The Lancet* (II), 552–5.

Salazar, L.M. *et al.* (1987). Costos de unidades del primer nivel de atención. In Funcionamiento de unidades de primer nivel de atención, unpublished mimeo. Centro de Investigaciones Multidisciplinarias en Desarrollo (CIMDER), Cali, Colombia.

Valle de Cauca (1980). *Proyecto para el diseño metodológico de educación continuada para promotoras de salud.* Servicio Seccional de Salud, Universidad del Valle, Cali, Colombia.

9 | Health volunteers in Sri Lanka

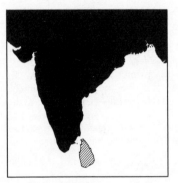

12 *Map of South Asia, with Sri Lanka highlighted. Drawn by Geoff Penna.*

Instead of community health workers, Sri Lanka has trained over 100,000 health volunteers who work part-time carrying out preventive and promotive activities in their communities. Why do they volunteer for this work? How effective are they? In this chapter we look in detail at health volunteers in four villages in Sri Lanka to try to answer these questions.

Although Sri Lanka is a poor country, its villagers are among the world's most educated. Free and accessible education for all for over forty years means that there are young men and women in relatively remote rural areas who have eleven or more years of schooling – the equivalent of their peers in the industrialized countries. The average age of marriage is also high. However, employment and further education opportunities are few, even for well-educated young people, so for many there is a considerable hiatus between the time of leaving school at about eighteen, and getting married at twenty-six. Does this explain why there are so many young health volunteers in Sri Lanka? In trying to answer this question we need to look at the context of the health volunteer programme.

Country background and socio-economic characteristics

The Democratic Socialist Republic of Sri Lanka, or Ceylon as it was known for many centuries, is a small island situated about 25 km from the southern tip of the Indian sub-continent.

It has a multi-ethnic and multi-religious population estimated in mid-1985 to number 15.9 million. The majority are Sinhalese (74 per cent), while the Indian and Sri Lankan Tamils make up 18.2 per cent of the population. The rest of the population is made up of Burghers, Moors, Malays and other ethnic groups. The religious mix reflects the ethnic pattern, with 70 per cent Buddhists, 15 per cent Hindus, 7.6 per cent Muslims and 7.5 per cent Christians. Political and racial tensions resulted in demands by Tamils for a separatist state in the North, and the country saw an escalation of violence during the 1980s. Attempts to resolve the conflict led to the establishment of an Indian 'peace-keeping' force in the North, and the formulation of a system of devolution of power. Fighting continued in the North, however, and spread rapidly to the South as the banned Janatha Vimukthi Peramuna (JVP, the People's Liberation Front) stepped up its destabilization of the state.

Despite Sri Lanka's poverty, with a per capita income of only US $340 in 1984, governments – before and since independence – have been committed to a number of important social welfare policies. Food was subsidized, education and health services were universal and free. These factors, among others, have been important in establishing a profile of high adult literacy (90 per cent males, 82 per cent females), late average age of marriage for females (twenty-five years), and low infant mortality and high life expectancy rates, as can be seen from Table 15. Sri Lanka's impressive achievements on the social front, however, were accompanied by relatively low rates of economic growth, and from the late 1950s the country faced continuous and chronic balance of payments problems.

Table 15 Demographic indicators, Sri Lanka, 1980–5.

Population (millions)	15.9
Population under 15 (%)	35.2
Population growth rate (%)	1.8
Crude birth rate (per 1000)	28.0
Crude death rate (per 1000)	6.1
Total fertility rate (births per women)	3.4
Life expectancy (males)	66.1
(females)	70.2
Infant mortality rate (per 1000 births)	23.1
Neonatal mortality (per 1000 births)	19.1

Sources: National census, 1981; Jayasuriya (1986); Unicef (1988)

In 1977 a new government, led by President Jayawardene, introduced a new set of economic policies with a heavy market orientation: price controls were abolished and subsidies were phased out. The economy grew steadily in the period from 1978 to 1984, with growth in a number of sectors including agriculture, construction, trade and transport. Domestic agriculture increased at about 5 per cent per annum, mainly due to a significant improvement in rice production that enabled the country to come close to self-sufficiency. Despite adjustment policies, however, Sri

Lanka's economy remained predominantly agricultural and service-orientated, with a thin and heavily import-dependent manufacturing sector. Since 1984 there has been a general slowing down in growth, as both foreign and domestic investors have adopted cautious attitudes towards investment because of the ethnic disturbances, and as international fluctuations in commodity prices and terms of trade have deteriorated (Unicef 1988).

One of the important aims of these economic strategies was to increase employment, and certainly unemployment as a percentage of the workforce dropped from a high of 24 per cent in 1973 to 11.7 per cent in 1981–2. However, unemployment remained extremely high in the age groups 14–18 years (30.8 per cent) and 19–25 years (28.8 per cent). Furthermore, 'Nearly 25% of those with GCE O levels and nearly 35% of those with GCE A levels are unemployed ... This high rate of educated unemployment is particularly significant for social and political stability' (Unicef 1988). This last statement has to be understood against the political landscape of Sri Lankan history. Universal franchise from 1931 established a highly politicized electorate, which averaged an 80 per cent turnout at national elections until the late 1980s, when deliberate harassment discouraged voting. The right-dominated United National Party, currently in power, took over from the left-orientated Sri Lankan Freedom Party in 1977, at a time when the economy was extremely depressed, and some six years after the violent youth insurgency of 1971. Post-1977 reforms were aimed at remedying the imbalances in the economy, as well as creating job opportunities for the educated youth of the country.

However, economic and racial tensions, which surfaced again in 1981, have continued to trouble Sri Lanka. The struggle for a separatist state by Tamil militants in the North has posed a serious threat to the unitary administration of the island. It remains to be seen whether the system of devolution being imposed in the country will provide a sustainable solution.

While the economic reforms followed since 1977 led to some economic growth, they also had some adverse effects on the welfare of vulnerable groups (Gunatilleke 1984). The policies resulted in high price increases, especially for food and kerosene. Despite substantial increases in investment in higher education, water supply, housing and health – financed to a large degree by foreign aid – expenditure on social services as a whole fell as a percentage of government expenditure, and acute malnutrition and inequalities increased (Gunatilleke 1987).

A number of post-1977 policies affected the health sector. The liberalization of imports of pharmaceuticals, for example, ended the state's monopoly to import drugs and led to an increase in drug consumption. Periodic shortages of drugs occurred at the PHC level of the government service, partly due to a doubling of the cost of basic drugs between 1979 and 1981 without a commensurate increase in budgetary provision. From 1977, government doctors previously not permitted to practise privately were allowed to do so, and while this increased accessibility to private care as they moved out of the cities, vacancies in government service, particularly preventive care services, became high (Unicef 1988).

Health and health services

The main health problems

Despite relatively good health indicators, some persistent problems reflect poverty and poor environmental conditions. While circulatory-system diseases are the leading cause of hospital deaths, complications of pregnancy and childbirth, and respiratory and infectious diseases are the commonest causes of morbidity (Table 16). The level of infectious and diarrhoeal diseases has not declined significantly since the mid-1960s, despite investments in water supplies and sanitation. Maternal mortality is 6 per 10,000 registered live births, and maternal, child and infant malnutrition and related diseases cause serious concern. While morbidity and mortality from malaria has declined there are signs of a possible growing insect resistance to the Malathion used in anti-malaria campaigns.

Table 16 Leading causes of hospital morbidity and mortality, Sri Lanka, 1985 (per 100,000 population).

	Cases	Deaths
Complications of pregnancy, childbirth and the puerperium	2719.3	1.1
Diseases of the respiratory system	2180.1	17.1
Infectious and parasitic diseases	2080.5	19.1
Injury and poisoning	1669.4	25.9
Diseases of the circulatory system	658.8	38.4
Diseases of the digestive system	613.0	8.4
Diseases of the genito-urinary system	610.5	3.1
Ill-defined conditions	1277.7	11.4

Source: Medical statistics division, Ministry of Health, 1986

The health system

Until 1983, all the country's health services, including the Ministry of Indigenous Medicine, were under the overall auspices of the Ministry of Health (MOH). In 1983, however, a new Ministry of Women's Affairs and Teaching Hospitals took over the administration of teaching hospitals, leaving the MOH responsible for all other services, both preventive and curative.

The government health services are organized in twenty divisions, each headed by a regional director of health services, and each of the divisions is sub-divided into 109 health areas. Each health area is organized into preventive services, headed by the medical officer of health, with a health team of public health inspectors, public health midwives who are sometimes referred to as family health workers, and public health nurses. The curative services are headed by the district medical officer who is in charge of the district hospital.

A health education and training component is included as a special programme under the MOH. The Health Education Bureau has a relatively autonomous position within the Ministry, with its own budget, building and vehicles. There are also a number of special vertical disease-control programmes, such as the anti-malaria campaign and the rabies control programme. Occupational services are provided independently by the government plantation sector for its own workers.

Overall, the government system provides a health facility within an average of 6 km of every household. There is wide variation in the quality of services offered, however, and because of good transport many patients bypass primary-level facilities in favour of tertiary-level facilities.

Alternative sources

The private allopathic services
The free health system provided by the state is supplemented by a private paid system. There are two aspects to this system. First, government doctors can practise privately outside state working hours. They use a network of private and state medical institutions to provide services to private patients. Second, there is the entirely private medical practitioner system which provides services ranging from outpatient care at private dispensaries to specialized treatment in private hospitals and nursing homes. The private doctors, estimated to number about 600, provide curative and family planning services. Some banks, large firms and corporations employ their own doctors to provide outpatient care for their employees.

The private indigenous sector
A second arm of the MOH is the Ministry of Indigenous Medicine, which functions under a separate minister and is responsible for training, research and dissemination of knowledge and of drugs.

The ayurvedic alternative to allopathic medicine, once a vibrant system, stagnated under colonial times. However, even in 1987 it had about 16,000 registered practitioners, plus a number of others who acquired knowledge through family tradition and who practise informally. The ayurvedic medical college and government hospital provide training, inpatient and outpatient medical care. A programme for the propagation of herbal gardens, and the use of herbal remedies for simple ailments, is being actively promoted by the Ministry of Indigenous Medicine.

Resources for health services

Social services expenditure by government fell from 33 per cent in 1977 to 22 per cent in 1983, and continued to fall in the later 1980s. Expenditure (both capital and recurrent) on health services also fell in the 1980s, till in 1985 it was 1 per cent of GNP and 4 per cent of total government expenditure (MOH 1985). Community health services suffered the greatest loss: 70 per cent of recurrent expenditure in the mid-1980s went to curative services, and of the 25 per cent spent on prevention, over half was on the vertical malaria-control programme. The ratio of capital to recurrent expenditure rose from 2.4 per cent in 1971–2 to over 50 per cent in 1983 (World Bank 1986). This reflects the huge capital expenditure on tertiary facilities, partly influenced by the availability of foreign aid. Around 70 per cent of capital expenditures for family planning in 1980 were externally financed (World Bank 1986).

Private expenditure on health almost matches state expenditure. One study suggested that private resources expended on health came to 910 million rupees (13 million US $) in 1982, while state-financed expenditure on health came to 1,309 million rupees (18.7 million US $) (WHO 1985).

Health personnel

The MOH estimates there are about 2,300 doctors in Sri Lanka (1 per 6,608 population), of whom about 1,700 are serving in government health facilities, mostly at the tertiary level. Most rural hospitals and dispensaries are staffed by assistant medical practitioners.

The most numerous health worker, and most peripheral, is the public health midwife (PHM), or family health worker. Each PHM covers a population of about 3,000, although actual coverage varies widely throughout the country. PHMs focus on home visiting for maternal and child health (MCH) activities, and, since most deliveries are done in institutions (79 per cent), do very few deliveries themselves. They also conduct antenatal and pre-school clinics, often in *ad hoc* community centres. From 1978 selection procedures for this cadre changed, and training was accelerated. Selection by a competitive examination was superseded by selection through a job bank containing the names of those who wanted a government job. To get onto the job bank list requires the patronage of a member of parliament. This has led to some tension between senior and junior PHMs, the former arguing that the latter are political appointees (Nichter 1986). It is commonly asserted that the newer PHMs are not as vocationally orientated as the older PHMs.

The development of the health volunteer programme

Voluntarism is a visible feature of life in Sri Lanka, possibly because of the influence of Buddhism. For a Buddhist, merit gained through good deeds is an important central concept. However, other circumstances have also affected the willingness to give voluntary service. The combination of Buddhism, with its emphsis on enlightenment which is easily identified with education, and a relatively autonomous female population (Caldwell 1986) – plus free education from the 1940s – established a relatively well-educated female population with few job opportunities. Voluntary work was seen as a legitimate activity for such (largely middle-class) women. By the 1970s education levels had also risen markedly in the rural villages, as had age of marriage, and, as we saw above, young men and women faced years after formal schooling with few employment opportunities. The demand for places on vocational courses or in higher education was thus far higher than the supply, and in such circumstances volunteering for health activities held some attraction. Furthermore, for many young unmarried women, voluntary work sanctioned them to move about in the community.

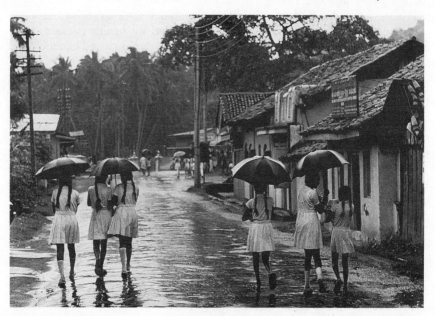

13 *Levels of female education are high, but employment opportunities are few and far between; volunteering for health activities holds great attraction. Photo: CWDE World Bank by Tomas Sennett.*

The involvement of school teachers and village and community leaders in voluntary work in public health activities can be traced as far back as 1915, to the Rockefeller Foundation-sponsored campaign for the control of hookworm infestation. Again, during the malaria epidemic of 1934–5 extensive involvement of voluntary workers was a special feature of the government's malaria-control programme. Non-governmental organizations began involving volunteers from the 1950s.

The main growth of the volunteer programme, however, began in the mid-1970s. International organizations such as Unicef introduced volunteers in urban slums (Adamson 1982), and the indigenous Sarvodaya Shramadana volunteer movement started in the 1950s and expanded in the 1970s. The latter involved volunteers working at village level in teaching and development projects, as well as health and nutrition. Another indigenous volunteer group was the Saukyadana movement which had health volunteers working in villages. Service organizations, such as the Family Planning Association, started to train volunteers in the 1970s, expanding from sixty in 1973 to 40,000 in 1987. Many other non-government agencies also supported small volunteer programmes: Oxfam, Save the Children (UK and US), SIDA and JOICFP, a Japanese organization.

The largest trainer of volunteers within government, however, is the Health Education Bureau, part of the Public Health Division of the MOH. The interest of the Health Education Bureau in a volunteer programme stemmed from two separate experiences. First, in the newly opened Mahaweli development areas, where settlers were being given land to farm, other services were few and far between. Health services were inaccessible and malaria incidence was high. Second, a United Nations Fund for Population Activities (UNFPA) family planning programme started in the early 1970s, with a relatively large component for communications. This became the responsibility of the Health Education Bureau, whose staff felt it important to tie family planning into other activities at village level, and to stress interpersonal communications. Harnessing the potential of educated young men and women in rural areas in order to provide continuity to the message and contact between the community and health staff was a strong motivation for training health volunteers. Thus volunteers were originally conceived as having a broad role. They were agents of development, spearheading community participation within their own communities, as well as educators and communicators. In this latter role, they were seen as assisting in the wider coverage of health services in areas where health staff were insufficient (Patrick 1978). They were never intended to be mere family planning motivators.

From 1976 the Health Education Bureau developed its volunteer programme, producing guidelines for health staff on selection procedures, teaching, and so on. In this they depended most heavily on PHMs, who came under the auspices of the Family Health Bureau, another section of the Department of Public Health within the Ministry of Health.

From a very early stage the PHM was an essential element in the health volunteer programme; success depended a great deal on her interest. Other health staff, such as the public health inspectors and regional health educators, were also important, but there were fewer of them. The PHM was expected to organize the selection of volunteers, explain the programme to the community, train the volunteers, and then provide supervision and support in order to sustain the programme. The volunteer programme therefore developed in patches, where there was interest and recognition of the potential value of the volunteers.

By the 1980s the Health Education Bureau had, through its enthusiasm and training programmes, persuaded sufficient health staff to start volunteer programmes that in 1987 it could claim that 100,000 volunteers had been trained in the decade since 1976. However, the volunteer programme is informal, with few responsibilities and relatively low expectations. It is difficult to get accurate figures on attrition rates or numbers of volunteers actively engaged. Thus, while the accepted official figure is 100,000 trained between 1976 and 1987, with attrition rates of 10 per cent per annum, this is an estimate based on the instructions to PHMs to train twenty volunteers per village, as we shall see below.

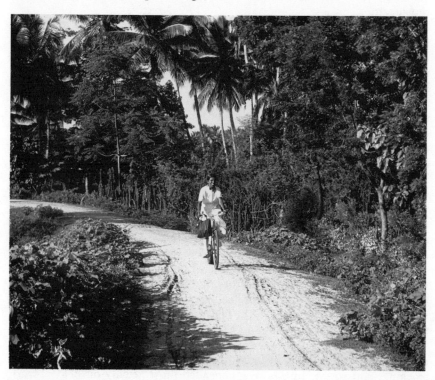

14 Public health midwives cycle or walk to visit households and health volunteers. Photo: Thierry Mertens (London School of Hygiene).

Training has so far taken place in 5,000 villages. Opinions differ on the current number of volunteers working regularly, with one conservative estimate being 18,000. The volunteer programme depends crucially on the PHM's energy and interest for both training and day-to-day contact with volunteers. There are no material incentives for either health staff or volunteers. This means the costs for the programme are extremely low, and the sustainability of the programme rests on contact with health staff, seminar programmes, health exhibitions, and so on, which only take place regularly in some areas. However, alternative methods of rewarding volunteers would carry huge cost implications, given the extent of their coverage. In the settlement areas of the Mahaweli scheme, where Unicef trains and equips health volunteers, it is estimated that training and equipment costs are about 200 rupees (US $5) per month per volunteer. There are altogether about 840 such volunteers trained in various sections of the Mahaweli scheme, so they are a small percentage of all the health volunteers trained.

Guidelines sent to all PHMs and public health inspectors by the MOH indicate that each field officer should train at least twenty volunteers to assist them in their community work. This activity was largely left to the health field-staff who were not directly responsible to the Health Education Bureau, while initiatives for training health volunteers did in fact rest primarily with the Health Education Bureau.

Demonstrable evidence of the success of health volunteer programmes in some areas (in helping health staff to establish links with the community and expand PHC activities to peripheral areas) moved the Minister of Health to recognize and acknowledge publicly the volunteer programme. From mid-1986 it was made clear that volunteers could be considered favourably for both PHM training and unskilled employment in hospitals or other Department of Health positions. Before this, MOH officials had always denied that being a volunteer could be considered as an opening to employment or training.

While these statements have marked a change in MOH policy, in the sense that volunteers are publicly recognized, the volunteer programme continues to be seen as informal and non-institutional. It was conceived as an informal community service when the PHC system was revised in 1980, and this has to be understood within the context of severe national budgetary constraints. Government economic policy has put pressure on public sector expenditure, which has led to a decline in funds for social services such as health and education.

Thus, while the MOH has acknowledged the value of the volunteer programme, it remains extremely cautious about formalizing it in any way, especially if any such policy change contains resource implications.

Volunteers in Anuradhapura district

In order to find out more about health volunteers, a small study was carried out in Anuradhapura district. Anuradhapura was one of the ancient capitals of Sri Lanka in the fifth century BC, situated in the dry zone of the country. It has no river, yet it was once the country's rice bowl. Cultivation was entirely by irrigation, which was provided by an intricate man-made system of reservoirs and channels (called tanks). The dry zone was neglected during colonial times, the tanks fell into disuse and became breeding grounds for malaria mosquitoes. Villages were abandoned.

In 1978 the Mahaweli River Accelerated Development scheme began to try to exploit the dry zone. By diverting water from the Mahaweli river it was planned to irrigate the area so that landless families could be given land, food production could be restored and hydro-electric power could be generated. By the early 1980s thousands of families had been moved into the Mahaweli settlement areas and had received two-and-a-half acres of land for a homestead and cultivation. New varieties of rice, techniques of cultivation and modern agrarian methods infused fresh vigour into what had been neglected rural areas. However, the newly released land was underdeveloped: there were few health or other social services, and the new settlers suffered from bouts of malaria.

Methodology of the study

The main aims of the Sri Lanka study were to examine the motivation of volunteers who were participating in the health volunteer programme introduced by the Health Education Bureau, and to see what sort of work they were doing and how far it was effective within the communities where they worked. The national study relied largely on published and unpublished reports from a series of sources, and on interviews with government officials involved in the programme, as well as with others from relevant non-governmental organizations.

The local-level study was carried out in two areas, and looked at the work of two different types of volunteer. In the settlement area (Mahaweli) the volunteers have some curative tasks, while in the non-settlement (non-Mahaweli) area, volunteers undertake purely educative and promotive activities. In each of the settlement and non-settlement areas one PHM catchment area was randomly selected, and then within each PHM area two villages were selected purposefully.

The research locations were all in Anuradhapura district, two villages in the Mahaweli system 'H' and two villages outside the Mahaweli area. Although quite close to each other (the furthest were 12 km apart) there were differences in the characteristics of the villages. None of the four villages was so affected by the political unrest as to be inaccessible to researchers who, having received a short training, lived in the areas continuously for a month, and visited frequently over a three-month period. Methods used included the following:

- questionnaires were completed by 136 health volunteers (69 in the settlement areas, 67 in the non-settlement areas) and 70 public health midwives in the two locations
- interviews were held with 120 householders in the four villages, as well as other health staff (medical officers of health, public health inspectors and health educators)

- in-depth interviews were held with 10 PHMs, 30 volunteers and 20 householders
- focus-group discussions were held with villagers in all four villages.

Profile of health volunteers

A total of 136 health volunteers were studied in the two research areas, 69 in the settlement areas and 67 in the non-settlement areas (see Table 17).

Table 17 Profile of health volunteers, Anuradhapura district, Sri Lanka.[1]

94% were female
76% were unmarried
78% were between 22 and 26 years
88% had GCE O levels or higher
65% had been volunteers for three or more years

[1] Average for settlement and non-settlement volunteers

Only 5 of the total were male. In the non-settlement areas, 69 per cent had been volunteers for over three years (62 per cent in the settlement areas).

In both settlement and non-settlement groups most of the health volunteers were between 22 and 26 years, as can be seen from Table 18.

Table 18 Age of health volunteers in the Sri Lanka study (per cent).

Age group (years)	Settlement areas N = 69	Non-settlement areas N = 67
17–21	19	16
22–26	49	57
27–31	19	16
32+	13	11
Total	100	100

The majority in this age group were unmarried: 82 per cent in the non-settlement areas, 70 per cent in the settlement areas. Access to free schooling was apparent in the large numbers of health volunteers who had had at least eleven years of schooling, many having taken the equivalent of the GCE O level examination. In the non-settlement areas, 94 per cent of volunteers had O levels or higher qualifications (83 per cent in the settlement areas).

How were volunteers introduced to the programme?

Although volunteers are supposed to be chosen by the community to which they are accountable, this seldom occurs. In both areas the majority of health volunteers stated they were recruited by health staff. In the non-settlement areas, 91 per cent had become health volunteers through their contact with the PHM (54 per cent in the settlement areas). In the settlement areas other health volunteers and family members persuaded 26 per cent of the health volunteers to take on the task. This method of selection was confirmed by the fact that 80 per cent of households did not know how volunteers were selected.

It is noteworthy that some volunteers have been involved in other volunteer programmes, such as the Family Planning Association. Many health volunteers were also simultaneously active in other voluntary activities: in the settlement areas 62 per cent, in the non-settlement areas 57 per cent. Indeed, in many families, both health volunteers and other family members were involved in other voluntary work, as is shown in Table 19.

Table 19 Involvement in other voluntary activities, Sri Lanka (per cent).

	Settlement N = 69	Non-settlement N = 67
Neither family members nor volunteers involved in other voluntary activities	4.3	7.5
Both family members and volunteers involved in other activities	59.4	44.8
Family members involved in other activities, but not volunteers	23.3	35.8
Health volunteers, but not family members involved in other voluntary activities	13.0	11.9
Total	100.0	100.0

The kinds of voluntary activity in which people engaged were varied, although it was notable that in a high proportion of families they were temple trustees – suggesting volunteers came from families with relatively high social status. Mostly, however, their parents (or in the case of married volunteers, their husbands) were farmers (71 per cent), with very few in professional occupations, such as teaching.

The tradition of voluntary activity is probably an important characteristic of health volunteers, demonstrating an involvement with the community in which they live. It does not exist among the PHMs: the questionnaire completed by PHMs revealed that 79 per cent had no involvement with community work or voluntary organizations, before or after becoming PHMs (other than their interactions with the community in the normal course of their health work). Of those who were now PHMs only 6 per cent had been health volunteers before training.

What motivates health volunteers to volunteer?

It was only in mid-1986, when the MOH announced that health volunteers with required qualifications would have preferential access to PHM training courses and jobs in the health department, that volunteering became a possible path to future employment. Sixty per cent of volunteers put their main reason for volunteering as the hope that this would lead to employment, and over half had already applied for jobs, although not always in the health sector.

However, more than a third put service to the community as their primary motivation for volunteering, and many volunteers gave multiple reasons which included self-improvement through further training. It seems that the material expectations from volunteering are by no means the only forces driving people to volunteer, and that satisfaction is gained from helping others, especially where – as in the settlement volunteers – they can offer material help: 'Officials come from outside and go away. We live here and see the hardships people undergo. They have to go 4–5 miles with a sick person sometimes. It is a great merit to relieve pain.'

Focus-group discussions with health volunteers confirmed another motive: that of liking to work outside their homes, to use otherwise idle time. As we have seen, the volunteer programme gives young women an opportunity to work in an area which gives them social recognition, legitimates their moving around the locality, and identifies them with relatively high-status health professionals.

Adequacy and relevance of volunteer training

Training was one of the main differences between settlement and non-settlement volunteers. Settlement volunteers have signs outside their houses, which say 'health volunteer supported by Unicef'. They receive a three-month course of training, and have a small number of medicines which they replenish on a once-per-month trip to a nearby health facility. They carry stocks of aspirin, oral rehydration solution (ORS) packets (from Unicef or manufactured locally), cicatrine for wounds and chloroquine and primaquine to treat malaria. These volunteers keep simple records, and during the malaria season may get ten or more people per day coming to them with fever, which is assumed to be malaria.

In contrast, the non-settlement volunteers have no medicines, receive a much shorter training (up to five days) and do not have a formal, regular meeting with health staff once a month. Although the Health Education Bureau has produced guidelines on volunteer training, it varies significantly from place to place. Much of the learning is done in formal lectures from health personnel, and less than half the non-settlement volunteers felt their training was adequate, while 63 per cent of settlement volunteers were satisfied with their training. Twenty per cent of non-settlement volunteers felt that they needed to be taught methods of communication, so that they could transmit health messages more easily. General feelings of inadequacy led volunteers to want more training: 'Often we have to go to the public health midwife to get an answer, and then tell the householder. When this happens they lose faith in us and refuse to accept any advice we give them.'

Householders themselves were more concerned with immediate, emergency treatment, and wanted health volunteers to have the ability to treat snake bites and wounds. Since, as we have seen, there is a plethora of different health services, indigenous and allopathic private practice as well as government services, in even quite rural areas, the emphasis on emergency treatment by householders is perhaps not surprising. Non-urgent ills can be taken to a number of alternative health-care providers, although the choice in the settlement areas is more limited.

The effectiveness of volunteers

Since most of the volunteers' tasks are educational (although settlement volunteers appear to spend most time on treatment), it is extremely difficult to measure their effectiveness. Although the Health Education Bureau's guidelines stipulate that base-line studies should be undertaken before training health volunteers, no base-line studies were available in the study areas. Much reliance had to be put on levels of knowledge (not always easy to check against behaviour), and attitudes.

In the settlement areas, volunteers were known by householders for their curative tasks, malaria treatment and first aid, rather than home visits or health education. However, the answers given during the research period coincided with Unicef's change in policy in that area, where up till recently most of the health volunteers had been male. Unicef's decision to insist on female volunteers had raised doubts in the communities' minds (expressed in the household interviews, focus-group discussions and in-depth dialogues), especially since many male volunteers had been replaced by their wives. Responses included doubts about the capacity and usefulness of these new (as yet untrained) volunteers. However, the value put on being able to get treatment for malaria during the malaria season was made clear, as was first aid for wounds acquired in the fields.

In the non-settlement areas, volunteers were clearly seen as advisers and educators, with no curative role. How effective were they? Judging from household interviews, a PHC package of messages was well known by most families. This comprised knowledge about family planning; supplementary feeding and weaning; boiling drinking water; use of latrines; the need for immunization; good nutrition, such as eating leafy vegetables; and malaria control.

Of course, the same messages were conveyed by the PHMs, but from questionnaires and records it was apparent that they could only complete visits to 40 per cent of the households for which they were responsible in the settlement areas, and 58 per cent in the non-settlement areas. Health volunteers, on the other hand, according to householders, visited homes regularly (72 per cent received a visit at least once a month), except for one settlement village where volunteers were rarely seen (only 13 per cent of these households received regular visits). While health volunteers may have played a part in imparting these messages, however, many other factors were also at play. In the settlement villages, 95 per cent of householders in one village had latrines, compared with 45 per cent in the other village. This was less due to the effects of health education than to the fact that one village was in a deforested, open area, and the other was surrounded by jungle. Similarly, although stated contraceptive use was high (65 per cent of households used some sort of modern contraceptive method, 32.5 per cent of whom had had tubectomies – which mirrors contraceptive prevalence rates of 62 per cent reported by the 1987 Demographic and Health Survey (Hettiarchi 1987), it is unclear whether health volunteers played any part in imparting knowledge or changing behaviour in this respect.

Patronage by health workers was seen to bring credibility to the health volunteers (and thus to improve the status of their knowledge in the eyes of the householders). Much, therefore, depended on the amount of contact they had with the PHMs or public health inspectors. The mean number of contacts between health volunteers and the PHM was 3.2 in a three-month period. According to the PHMs, 74 per cent of them took health volunteers on visits to households, either sometimes or often, and they sometimes relied on health volunteers to call at homes they could not visit. In one deprived village the PHM relied heavily on health volunteers because caste considerations made it difficult for her to visit homes. In this particular area health volunteers were noted by the PHM to be dedicated and active in helping the community. Health volunteers also assisted in the twice-monthly clinics.

According to household questionnaires nearly all homes (84 per cent) with children under five years had been visited by the PHM in the six months before the interview. PHMs (in these areas anyway) appeared to be able to meet some of their 'at-risk homes' targets, if not to visit all homes. Another study of over 3,000 pregnant women in three districts found that PHMs had made home visits to only approximately half the mothers during pregnancy (Meegama and Gaminiratne 1986). However, it was also clear from focus-group and in-depth discussions that some households were visited more frequently than others, for social rather than for primarily professional reasons. In one village the household of a bank employee had received eighteen visits from the PHM in the previous three months, yet this family used a private practitioner instead of the clinic for preventive and curative care.

Perceptions of volunteer roles and functions

In trying to assess the roles of health volunteers it is impossible to separate the different factors that affect their work. From the qualitative data it is clear that sheer personality, capability and enthusiasm play a major role.

The links with the health services are important in legitimizing and giving credibility to the volunteer's role, and much depends on the interest and number of contacts health volunteers have with PHMs. We have seen that these vary considerably. Some PHMs do not value the volunteers, and clearly this attitude would affect their relationships with them. Asked whether volunteers would still have a role to play if there were sufficient midwives, 67 per cent of the PHMs said 'no'. It appeared that some PHMs had had unfortunate contacts with volunteers, and felt volunteers tried to emulate them. Sometimes they saw them as a threat to their authority and acceptance by the community, and some complained that 'do-gooding' attitudes of volunteers led to disregard of the PHMs' instructions. Those PHMs who saw health volunteers not as stopgaps, but in a wider role, perceived them to be performing tasks that PHMs were not able to do well: conveying information or urgent messages, understanding, knowing and communicating with the community. However, many PHMs saw volunteers as useful adjuncts to their own work: assisting PHMs with their visits and in the clinics, notifying emergencies, telling villagers of clinic dates, and bringing people to the clinic — all these were tasks PHMs valued in the health volunteers. They clearly saw volunteers as extra pairs of hands in health service activities and there was very little indication that broader, development tasks were considered part of the volunteers' roles.

Householders' views on volunteers were mixed. In some areas they were highly appreciated, partly because they gave a personal service: looking after the home and children while the mother took a child to the clinic; administering ORS to a child with diarrhoea; assisting at the clinic. However, 30 per cent of households did not know what the health volunteers did, and some considered them insufficiently qualified.

Health volunteers themselves showed some lack of confidence. In interviews they made comments such as: 'People are afraid to follow our advice. We are at home so they think we don't know anything'; 'Elderly people don't need our advice. They believe in traditions, in superstitions. We do not know enough to convince them'. Certainly, some volunteers mentioned the difficulty of persuading people to follow allopathic rather than folk practices, and were confused by their training which emphasized the former, and their experience, which continually encountered the latter. They found themselves caught between the community members' custom of using certain herbs and leaves for wounds, skin rashes, worms and scabies and the often negative attitudes of the professional health staff to these methods. Not having drugs (and being reluctant to use traditional methods) some health volunteers, particularly in the non-settlement areas, had resorted to buying certain preparations, simply to 'keep faith' with the community. In one of the research areas, health volunteers had bought cicatrine (for dressing wounds).

Finally, health volunteers felt another sense of dissonance between their training and their experience. Training courses focused on allopathic responses to preventive and curative activities specifically related to health.

But their communities had a much more holistic view of health in which, when asked about their health problems, householders talked of roads, stagnant and insufficient water, absence of nursery schools, of latrines and of first aid. In the settlement areas male health volunteers were more valued than the females who replaced them because they were seen to be more capable of solving these general problems through their involvement in village organizations, their access to officials, and so on.

In spite of these difficulties, many health volunteers claimed that volunteering had changed their lives: 75 per cent felt they had gained personally – they were more aware of health, had obtained new knowledge and had learned the value of team work: 'Idling at home after school was mentally depressing. Now I am part of society, mentally and physically revived.' They also used words such as 'improvement', 'progress', 'maturity', 'unselfish', 'respect of villagers', 'acting in an emergency', to describe their satisfaction with their roles.

In summary, health volunteers are young, single, well-educated and usually female. In this study (although the numbers are small) 65 per cent had had three or more years' experience as volunteers, so although attrition rates were quite high, a core of regular volunteers sustained the programme. There were few differences in outlook between the settlement and non-settlement volunteers, although their training and activities differed. An important characteristic of health volunteers is that the majority participate in other voluntary organizations. In spite of a strong voluntary experience, however, the driving force for health volunteering is the prospect of future employment or training. In terms of effectiveness it is difficult to separate the effects of volunteers from other influences. However, of the households interviewed, 65 per cent had a latrine, 84 per cent had had their houses sprayed with Malathion and 65 per cent of children under two years were fully immunized, according to their health cards. It is likely that volunteers had some effect on these figures, although this would vary considerably from area to area, and even from volunteer to volunteer.

Conclusions

It is extremely difficult to assess the health volunteer programme. Its informality, decentralized training and control, and the paucity of statistics available characterize both its strengths and weaknessess. Although it was originally conceptualized as a broad development programme, with volunteers spearheading change in their villages, it has become an adjunct to the services offered by the PHM. How far this is a concern is not clear: much value is put on the volunteers' health service roles.

While some downplay attrition rates – arguing that a short training costs very little and has a mass education effect – there is still a loss of potential, and although low, the opportunity costs of PHMs' and public health inspectors' time for training and supervising remains a cost to the health service. By taking a few simple steps the volunteer programme could be strengthened to make it more effective. For example, incentives could be devised that would encourage volunteers to stay on. These need not be too costly: many volunteers mentioned how much they valued the training they received. Building in a continuing education series may be incentive enough to retain an active volunteer. Setting targets or projects, asking for assistance in monitoring and evaluation, are all helpful in providing guidelines for work and goals to work towards.

A more radical approach would be to monitor the rate at which volunteers receive preferential places on midwifery training courses. If the numbers of volunteers gaining entry to these courses is small, the MOH could consider adopting a policy of positive discrimination in favour of health volunteers without the necessary qualifications but with proven dedication and experience. Guidelines for such criteria would need to be carefully drawn up and, possibly, a special examination devised. Such a recruitment policy would have the advantage of creating a community- and vocationally-orientated cadre of PHMs, which is not the case at present. However, any such alteration of the necessary educational requirement for PHM training would undoubtedly meet with resistance from PHMs, and would probably therefore only be cautiously considered by the Ministry of Health.

References

Adamson, P. (1982). The gardens. *New Internationalist*, 109, 7–28.

Caldwell, J. (1986). Routes to low mortality in poor countries. *Population and Development Review*, 12, 2, 171–80.

Gunatilleke, G. (1984). Health and development in Sri Lanka. Paper delivered to the Inter-regional seminar on health for all, 26 August–7 September 1984, sponsored by UNDP, UNICEF and WHO. Colombo.

Gunatilleke, G. (1987). *Children in Sri Lanka*. Marga Institute/Unicef, Colombo.

Hettiarchi, S. (1987) Fertility levels of Lankan women have declined. *Daily News*, Colombo, 25 September.

Jayasuriya, R. (1986) Use of indicators in monitoring and evaluation of national strategies for health for all: experience of Sri Lanka. *World Health Statistics Quarterly*, 39, 4, 298–310.

Meegama, S.A. and Gaminiratne, K.H.W (1986). *Perinatal and Neonatal Morality – Some Aspects of Maternal and Child Health in Sri Lanka*. Dept of Census and Statistics/Unicef, Colombo.

Ministry of Health (1985). *Health Bulletin*. Colombo.

Nichter, M. (1986). The primary health centre as a social system: PHC, social status and the issue of team-work in South Asia. *Social Science and Medicine*, 23, 4, 347–55.

Patrick, W. (1978). *The Volunteer Health Worker in Sri Lanka*. Health Education Series 4, Health Education Bureau. Colombo.

Unicef (1988). Sri Lanka: the social impact of economic policies during the last decade. In Cornia, G.A. Jolly, R. and Stewart, F. (eds), *Adjustment with a Human Face*, Vol 2, Clarendon Press, Oxford.

WHO (1985). National study on resource allocation for MCH-FP in Sri Lanka. Maternal and Child Health Unit, Division of Family Health. Unpublished report MCH/85.7. WHO, Geneva.

World Bank (1986). Sri Lanka: health and family planning sector report. Unpublished report by Population, Health and Nutrition Department, World Bank, Washington DC., mission carried out in 1983.

PART IV

Conclusions

10 | Just another pair of hands?

What conclusions can we draw about national community health worker (CHW) programmes? Elsewhere we have argued that they are in crisis not because the concept of CHWs is incorrect, but because the support and supervision that make them effective are all too often missing (Walt 1988). Is this a fair analysis and, if so, what implications does this conclusion have? We try here to answer this question within the structure we outlined in Parts I and II of this book. First, we examine the context within which implementation of national CHW programmes has occurred, then we look at each of the central issues: the definition of a CHW; the tasks and skills of CHWs; CHWs as links in the health system; and the sustainability of national CHW programmes.

The context of implementation

The Alma Ata meeting on primary health care (PHC) in 1978 was an international initiative promoting a revolutionary shift in health policy. It was based on a decade of cumulated experience and changing ideas in which a technical agency (WHO), committed to the eradication of disease, joined with a development agency (Unicef) to promote the affirmation that improvements in health were caused by economic, social and political changes and were not merely the outcome of the work of existing health services. The principles which formed the basis of the approach were equity, intersectoral collaboration, community involvement, emphasis on prevention, and appropriate technology. CHW programmes were in many ways seen as encompassing all these principles: *equity* by extending services to neglected populations; *intersectoral collaboration* by working with other sectors' community workers and indigenous practitioners, and including tasks traditionally seen as beyond the health sector (such as water and sanitation); *community involvement* by their close links with communities via selection and accountability; *prevention* through the definition of their tasks; and *appropriate technology* because CHWs were from the communities where they worked and could be trained locally and rapidly.

Unfortunately, however, the PHC approach was launched at a time of major economic change. Within three years of the Alma Ata meeting the world economy was experiencing the most severe and prolonged recession since the 1930s. Seventy per cent of developing countries suffered from negative cumulative growth rates in the 1980s (Unicef 1988). In their attempts to re-create conditions for growth, control inflation and reduce debt, the major international finance organizations, such as the International Monetary Fund and the World Bank, forced a good number of developing countries to introduce adjustment policies. In many cases these policies exacerbated poverty and depressed employment and real incomes. Some countries performed better than others, but by the end of 1984 average gross domestic product per capita in Latin America and the Caribbean had fallen back to the level of 1976. The situation in the sub-Saharan countries remains especially bleak – by 1983 income per capita was about 4 per cent below the level of 1970 (Abel-Smith 1986). The impact of the Acquired Immune Deficiency Syndrome (AIDS) is as yet unknown, but predictions for African cities, in particular, are alarming. The combination of an increase in resistance to falciparum malaria, and continuing food insecurity, heralds grave consequences for health on this continent.

In many countries, economic recession in the 1980s has been accompanied by a growth in political instability, low-intensity warfare, and refugee and displaced-person migration. CHWs in rural areas have often been caught in the midst of horrendous levels of social, economic and political insecurity, and in some countries have been selected as targets by right- or left-wing military or revolutionary forces, or – as in the case of Mozambique – pure banditry. Within this period there has also been an ideological shift in many government policies that formerly supported collective, state action in health and education, to those which are increasingly promoting individual, private responsibility and encouraging a greater role for the private market, even in health. The attempt to diminish the role of the state in favour of private forces is being strongly led by the international financial institutions whose level of influence on national policy-making has increased as the recession has worsened and countries have been forced to increase their borrowing. The concrete effects of this situation are reflected in decreased budgets available for the health sector (Abel-Smith 1986) and increased reliance on donors for both preventive programmes and recurrent funding. This has further skewed national policies towards donor-led interests which from the early 1980s have tended towards more selective, almost vertically organized programmes, such as those of immunization and oral rehydration (Rifkin and Walt 1986).

The change from the relatively buoyant economic and political climate of the 1970s when PHC was launched, to the depression of the 1980s, has had profound implications for the implementation of the PHC approach. The two international agencies most involved in PHC were led during this period by devoted activists – Halfdan Mahler at WHO and James Grant at Unicef – who, each in his own style, promoted the change in health policy towards the PHC approach more decisively and forcefully than any previous leaders had ever done with past policies. Other international donors, as well as non-governmental organizations, and indeed, member countries, soon accepted the persuasive arguments in favour of PHC. The result was that, very often, enthusiasm and haste triumphed over planning and management. The desire for measurable outcomes led to an emphasis on selective interventions rather than support for the steady development of comprehensive PHC. CHW programmes were introduced rapidly as a demonstration of countries' commitment to PHC. The expansion of health services, started in the 1970s, was difficult to sustain in this climate, and what began to suffer was the periphery.

Governments are more likely to be sensitive to demands from urban populations, where the effects of adjustment policies may end in demonstrations and rioting. Furthermore, the demands for upgrading – or building new – hospitals and health centres in cities and towns, many of which have seen unprecedented levels of growth in the last few decades, put even greater pressure on ministries of health to allocate ever scarcer resources to these ends. Such decisions may have huge 'knock-on' effects. Professional nursing staff may be attracted to the new institutions, and be even less willing to work in rural areas. The costs of equipment and drugs will rise, and what is likely to suffer is the primary level of care.

The political and economic climate as we enter the 1990s is gloomy, particularly in Africa. If realistic policies are to be adopted this has to be taken into account when thinking about national CHW programmes of the future.

Definitions: who is the community health worker?

There is a great diversity in national CHW programmes, but some generalizations can be made. From the three case-study countries, it is clear that the great majority of their CHWs are locally resident women, in their twenties or thirties. In Sri Lanka they have not yet married; in Colombia and Botswana they are single-parent families, relying on their own earnings. The lack of employment opportunities in rural areas plays an important part in attracting people to the role of CHW, even in Sri Lanka where they are unpaid but hope that volunteering will lead to a paid job. In Botswana, Colombia and Jamaica, all salaried programmes, this is borne out by the fact that attrition rates are low. The lack of employment opportunities also probably largely explains why some national programmes (for example, India and Zambia) have been, or continue to be, dominated by males.

The main characteristic that sets salaried CHWs apart from other health workers is that they cannot be transferred: they are (in theory) selected by the community and are representative of it, and so cannot be moved to another community as a CHW. However, even these differences between CHWs and other primary-level workers are beginning to be challenged in some countries. In practice, selection is seldom by community members, and in Botswana – and a few other places – an active decision has been made to transfer CHWs from one place to another.

While, in fact, the above similarities between programmes exist, the many differences should not be ignored. The length of time spent on training varies considerably – from five days in Sri Lanka, to four months in Botswana. In Colombia, CHWs have largely preventive tasks in people's homes; in Botswana similar tasks are carried out, but mostly in health facilities. CHWs in Sri Lanka, village communicators in Thailand, and many of the kaders in Indonesia, have only health education tasks, and work part-time, whereas in Colombia, Botswana and Jamaica they are full-time, relatively well paid, and have uniforms and pension rights. There are also those who fall between these two groups, such as the Thai volunteers and the Indian guides who receive honoraria rather than salaries, the Peruvian health promoters who are permitted to make a profit from selling drugs, or the Zambian village health workers who receive a small number of drugs to use for treatment.

Is it correct, therefore, to call both the health promoters of Colombia and the family welfare educators of Botswana community health workers? Ironically, in relation to the tasks they do, the most similar worker in Sri Lanka is the public health midwife (PHM) rather than the volunteer. The main difference is that the Sri Lankan PHM is trained for at least eighteen months, has higher-level educational qualifications and is transferable. Others have asked whether it would not be more correct in Botswana to call the traditional midwives the CHWs, rather than the actual family welfare educators (Anderson and Staugård 1988), because the traditional midwives are so clearly differentiated from the health services and are so much part of the community.

This diversity in the types of national CHW programme represents very little difference in expectations of what the workers will achieve: they are all expected to be extenders of health services, bridging gaps between fixed health facilities and local communities. Any conception of CHWs having developmental goals, or playing roles as change agents, remain occasional lapses of rhetoric. This is, of course, much less true in small, non-governmental programmes.

How then, should national programmes proceed? Instead of seeking to maintain the global definition of a CHW across all countries and within all parts of a country, it is important for both donors and governments to be more flexible. A clear distinction must be made between paid and volunteer workers. In particular, the differences in loyalty and working patterns (and thus, likely achievements) between health workers who are paid, and who therefore have strong ties to the health services and its professionals, and those who are unpaid volunteers, who work as CHWs of their own volition (even if this is motivated by a desire for eventual employment), must be recognized.

Greater flexibility implies looking at other forms of CHW programme. For example, the experiments in social mobilization, using volunteers who take part in major health drives once or twice a year (Unicef 1986; 1987) have been successful in attracting wide support and interest in particular issues over short periods. Such an approach addresses specific needs and may be more sustainable than expecting volunteers to work part-time or long-term. What the CHW is and does must reflect the circumstances (needs, resources) in which any CHW programme develops. For example, in some countries there are many private health care providers, including Western-trained doctors, herbalists, traditional midwives and drug sellers. In such situations, the introduction of a rapidly trained CHW may not add much to the choice or quality of care for the population (especially where support and supervision are fragile). As circumstances vary between different parts of a country it may be important for ministries of health to allow local initiatives to develop, even if this results in a variety of CHWs within one country. Decentralization – another concept which was much promoted in the health sector in the 1980s – should allow local health authorities to decide on how, and whether, a particular district can support CHWs. This is likely to lead to more realistic and appropriate planning for both training and supervision. Local health authorities might even decide to discontinue an existing programme in order to put more resources into supporting their primary level of the health service.

One of the arguments against allowing local authorities to develop their own programmes is that this could lead to inequity, with wealthier areas more likely to be able to support a CHW programme. There is evidence that this occurred in China. A national government concerned with equity has the opportunity to devise policies that allocate resources differentially to areas, depending on criteria that attempt to assess levels of need. Positive discrimination in resource allocation can, at least theoretically, overcome regional inequities. What is clear is that there is little point in insisting on uniformity in programmes when there is very little uniformity between geographical areas and even infrastructures within those areas. Through flexible funding practices, donors could assist in marginal areas.

Moreover, it is important not to see CHWs as the solution to establishing effective community participation, but rather to assess their role within an overall discussion of how to achieve community involvement. Being over-optimistic about the CHWs' role will only undermine their potential contribution. Questions of community participation go far beyond the health sector and are concerned with the democratic and cultural history of the state, the strength of its popular movements, and its present mechanisms – and tolerance – for community involvement.

It is likely that existing CHWs (especially those who are full-time government employees) will always be primarily accountable to the government. They are extenders of the health service. This situation need not be viewed negatively – both health professionals and communities are largely supportive of the very restricted role (compared with the global concept) played, for example, by CHWs in Botswana. In this role, CHWs have great potential for improving the coverage of the health services, but much depends on the attitudes of the professional primary-care staff, and the extent to which they, in turn, are supported. What is important is that community members know what CHWs are able to do and how their services can be obtained, which was not always the case in the countries that we studied.

Tasks and skills: what can community health workers do?

It is clear from this study that if CHWs do not have curative tasks and access to drugs they are not greatly valued by community members, and their preventive work is undermined. But where CHWs can give treatment, they then tend to divert most attention to it, and since the supervisors of CHWs are almost always clinically orientated nurses this tendency is exacerbated. The CHWs' work becomes almost completely confined to the health sector, and few intersectoral links are made except through a CHW's individual membership of voluntary organizations.

One of the difficulties of dividing time between preventive and curative tasks is this tendency to verge towards the latter. This is becoming apparent in Colombia where, although home visiting is theoretically the CHW's main activity and clear routines are established, the average number of visits per day was only four.

In Botswana, too, there has been a noticeable increase in time spent within health facilities. As one of the main reasons for training CHWs in Botswana was that they should spend time in the community, it is important to note how few homes actually receive visits. Family welfare educators spend less than 15 per cent of their working time on home visits, which last less than thirty minutes. It was clear that, almost from the beginning of the programme, home visiting had taken second place to health-facility work. An evaluation in Jamaica suggested that, in spite of grave shortages of CHWs, a high proportion remain based in clinics (Ennever *et al.* 1988). In Sri Lanka volunteers had responsibility for ten or so households that, on the whole, were very close to where they lived. It was, therefore, difficult to quantify the number and purpose of the visits because they were often extremely informal.

Establishing an effective balance between curative and preventive care is inextricably bound up, then, with the balance between the need for facility-based activities and home visits. In Botswana, an examination of fourteen clinics revealed that it was feasible to release CHWs from clinical duties to spend more time in the community, except in the busiest facilities. However, whether home visiting would be a more appropriate and effective way of improving health care (assuming CHWs would undertake increased visiting) than facility-based work, remains open to question. Immunization coverage rates, for example, are relatively high in most parts of Botswana, and, in order to increase them further, CHWs would have to visit target homes to persuade families to take children to health clinics. The feasibility of doing this – it may be difficult for CHWs for status or cultural reasons – has to be considered when optimizing CHW time. It may be better to hold more outreach clinics, run by professional primary-level staff, assisted by CHWs. However, it is certainly claimed that in some areas of Sri Lanka, door-to-door persuasion by health volunteers increased immunization coverage rates dramatically.

Ultimately the decision about the balance of care provided by CHWs must reflect the accessibility of other sources of care, and the acceptability and costs of providing them with wider clinical skills and the necessary drugs and supplies. However, this is inextricably tied up with concerns about the quality of the care CHWs are able to give. In theory they could probably undertake to do more than they are allowed: using simple diagnostic procedures, they could assess, for example, whether a child needs antibiotics (Ronsmans *et al.* 1988; Cherian *et al.* 1988); in Jamaica they take blood pressure to help identify hypertensives (Ennever *et al.* 1988). However, the quality of their care depends to a large extent on their receiving appropriate professional support and supervision. Where this is lacking, as is so often described, quality of care is unlikely to be high. Nevertheless, even with existing constraints on support, much could be done. For example, the CHWs' preventive and home-visiting role could be strengthened by clearer job descriptions, improved guidelines on what to do during home visits, better work scheduling, and the targeting of specific families who are most at risk. The more closely this is done with primary-level professional health staff, the better. Good management techniques are needed throughout the system.

The value of CHWs' having only promotive or educative tasks must remain an open question. From previous studies, there seems little likelihood of CHWs' being able to effect changes in behaviour that demand major changes in people's belief patterns or day-to-day activities. Only small changes are possible, such as persuading someone to take a child to an immunization session, or to undertake a clean-up campaign. The fact that CHWs are usually only volunteers, working part-time, lends further limitations. Not only may their efforts be relatively ineffective, but retaining their interest in the work may be difficult, as is borne out by the high attrition rates in CHW programmes. A lack of incentives, coupled with the likelihood of negative results, may serve to demoralize volunteers. And while it may be true that a volunteer programme's main goal is mass education, so that attrition rates are relatively unimportant, it is difficult to assess the outcome of such a programme over the short term.

In the final analysis, there is nothing to fault an attempt to give workers with relatively little education some basic skills so that they can help their own communities. Historically, this is the way that most professionals started – as apprentices learning from those already in practice for some time. What is different in national CHW programmes is that CHWs are not apprenticed to a specific professional. They are rapidly trained, often in classrooms far removed from the realities they face, and they do not have a mentor or teacher by their side to reinforce their learning by example. The supervision and support which should be more or less continual is missing. How can this be improved?

Community health workers as links in a chain

Existing weaknesses in support and management prompt the question whether it is worth having CHWs at all if they are not well supervised. Trained for short periods, lacking in confidence, armed with few tasks and skills, CHWs more than any other health worker need the backing of the health service. Yet this is an area of acknowledged weakness in all national programmes.

One of the main problems identified in the three case studies was that CHWs did not always know who their supervisors were: in Botswana many thought it was the clinic-orientated enrolled nurses, instead of the community health nurses (CHNs). In Sri Lanka all depended on the interest of the PHM or public health inspector. In Colombia CHWs complained of the high rates of turnover of supervisory staff who often did their one-year compulsory social service in a rural area and rarely stayed longer. Supervision itself was often weak: CHWs tended to get drawn into activities with nursing staff, not as learners but as extra pairs of hands. Continuing education opportunities were limited.

Weak health service support and management could perhaps be counteracted by community support. However, although community members in many countries express some appreciation of their CHWs and a certain degree of satisfaction with their services, any other community support is largely passive. In Botswana, where there were health committees in many villages, the relationship between committee members and CHWs was not usually vibrant and, with few exceptions, health committees have largely been inactive and therefore not a source of support for CHWs. This reflects a general problem affecting many committees imposed on communities: their members seldom understand their role, and initial enthusiasm degenerates rapidly into passivity.

How to deal with this problem of inadequate supervision and support is perhaps the greatest challenge facing national CHW programmes. Trying to establish national norms, except at a relatively general level, is probably counter-productive; allowances must be made for local flexibility because of variations in geographical area, transport and communications, the placement of fixed health facilities, numbers of staff available, and so on. Getting CHWs together may be a better solution for supervisors than trying to reach remote villages themselves. There are many instances of CHWs who are prepared to walk great distances every month or so in order to attend a meeting, receive a salary or restock with medicines. Some of these examples are heroic, such as the CHWs in Mozambique who brave the aggressive counter-revolutionary bands roving the countryside in order to reach district or provincial towns to restock on both drugs and learning. Regularity and quality of contact are both goals which could be met more often than they are at present.

However, all this necessitates changes in the attitudes and training of those who become supervisors. National policy-makers and donors need to take into account the costs of supervision, and make allowances for the payment to the supervisors of per diems where necessary, or time-off in lieu for visits to remote parts of a region. Regular meetings of CHWs should be given financial support so that at the very least refreshments are available, and bus fares (or other transport costs) can be met immediately. This is often difficult for local government systems to manage, and is an acknowledged weakness at district level in a great number of countries. Sometimes non-governmental organizations can be useful in meeting minor costs such as these, as well as helping support opportunities for regular continuing education. Almost all CHWs are hungry for more learning, and more than willing to attend refresher courses. It is the opportunities that are missing.

A system of supervision that improves quality of contact is important, too, and in many countries more training along these lines is required. Needless to say, much depends on the outlook of the supervisors. If they are essentially clinically orientated, their support for CHWs is likely to be focused on treatment skills, and their concern will be with individuals and families, and not with the community as a whole. PHNs or CHNs tend to be few in number and, while less clinically orientated than other nurses, may see their role largely limited to preventive activities such as antenatal and immunization clinics, and the follow-up of tuberculosis or leprosy patients. In many poor countries such nurses may also be called upon to distribute food. It is not surprising, then, if CHWs are expected to pursue similar activities, and that supervision and support are seen to be met if CHWs are involved in routine tasks in health facilities.

The ideal to strive for would be good management support and supervision for all peripheral services. CHW supervision needs to become a more thorough and detailed activity, a form of evaluation, and not an infrequent chore. For example, supervisors could spend two to three days each month with a group of CHWs, living with them in their villages. They should utilize checklists for supervision that include some notion of the quality of community encounters, and they should be trained in holding group discussions with community members. Contact between CHW and supervisor should be part of continuing education.

Clear policies on work scheduling, and realistic targeting of activities would also help supervision and support. Improved reward systems would boost CHW morale. These need not necessarily entail direct payment of CHWs: refresher courses or other types of training, or regular meetings, may be sufficient reward in themselves. Greater involvement in monitoring and evaluation or setting targets may also increase satisfaction, as well as achieve programme goals.

For example, much more could be done to interest supervisors in the use of information systems and surveys, so that supervision could become a process with an achievable and changing goal. Relatively simple household surveys to find out whether community members have used the available services – and if not, why not – may help to orientate both clinic and community work. Assessing coverage of immunizations, for example, could begin with existing records and census data. Supervisors working alongside CHWs doing such surveys or using information or records that already exist, and discussing the findings with them, would not only be teaching and reinforcing learning but would be giving a concrete goal to reach by which to measure progress. Motivation and interest in work is much more likely to be sustained with such an approach. However, this implies that supervisors themselves must be given good, practical field training in the use of such methods, and have the confidence to introduce them in their own areas. They will also need incentives to reinforce both training and experience, as well as to sustain their interest. New approaches are needed in thinking about non-financial incentives – for example, career structures that reward supervisory responsibilities, and professional meetings that provide a forum for discussion on field experience and research.

We have seen that CHWs are links in a chain, providing the bridge between primary-level services and community members. They cannot, however, be considered separately from primary-level services, for many of the weaknesses of support and supervision that have been noted in CHW programmes are, in fact, a feature of the entire peripheral level of the health service. Here supervision is often poor, stocks may be resupplied irregularly, and staff feel neglected. Poor management of health services is noted, time after time, in the staff lassitude that stems from low morale, and in the confusion that arises from unclear job descriptions or differentiation between jobs. The results may be witnessed in conflict and disharmony between staff, or between staff and community, or in disillusionment and even corruption, with pilfering or illegal private practice taking place quite openly.

In other words, improving support and supervision for national CHW programmes can only take place if it is considered within the framework of the whole health service. It is not possible to change support and supervision without looking at some of the above issues, and the relationships between the different levels of the infrastructure. However, instead of attempting to do this at a national level, local health authorities should be encouraged to find local solutions, facilitated with resources from national or central authorities. Local initiatives that encourage and support appropriate supervision may draw on resources available locally but not nationally.

Sustaining community health worker programmes

Where CHWs are paid, the main costs of programmes are salaries (possibly up to 90 per cent of costs). Training, supervision and management, including drugs and supplies, are much less, although altogether these costs can be substantial. For example, the cost of a home visit by a Colombian health promoter was twice the cost to the health service of an outpatient contact with a doctor. Even though the cost of this visit to the household was clearly much less, home visiting even by low-paid CHWs is, for the health services, relatively expensive.

It is clear that financial constraints have affected both the Botswana and Colombia programmes, since training has been effectively frozen in Colombia and fewer family welfare educators than originally envisaged are being trained in Botswana. The financing problems of the health sector as a whole suggest that there are obvious policy gaps between stated support for CHWs and likely future financial support. Ministry of health budgets in Sri Lanka and Colombia are highly skewed towards secondary or tertiary care. Similarly, the production of health personnel in Colombia heavily favours doctors, the most expensive cadre. And in Botswana, as in many other countries, little or no capital expenditure on the main hospitals during the 1970s has resulted in the need for substantial expenditure now – further skewing health expenditure patterns away from preventive care. How realistic is it, then, to expect the ministry of health to support salaried CHWs at the primary level in sufficient numbers to work efficiently in relatively remote or scattered populations? Donors will usually finance CHW training but it is unlikely that they will get involved in any long-term expenditure on recurrent costs. Is it more realistic to train CHWs who work only part-time, but who do not expect a salary?

While volunteer programmes appear much less expensive, especially where training is local and rapid, experience suggests that they are only feasible under certain conditions. This approach relies on substantial numbers of relatively well-educated men and women in rural areas, for whom training and employment opportunities are few. Religious and ethical values of serving others through voluntary work may also be a strong motivating force, as is seen in some Buddhist countries (for example, Burma, Sri Lanka and Thailand), and traditional authoritarian structures may also increase voluntarism, as in Indonesia. Political commitment, sometimes under adverse conditions, may also unite and stimulate voluntary effort, as witnessed in Nicaragua, for example. However, it is a myth that volunteer programmes are cheap – especially if run on a large scale – because high attrition rates result in substantial costs from the frequent training courses that are needed. The costs of support, supervision and supplies may also be large, especially if low activity rates are to be avoided.

Overall, it is essential that governments should set the problem of CHW financing within the wider debate about health-care financing, because it arises out of the sector-wide resource constraints. Failure in the past to plan for CHWs within PHC must not be continued in current and future financing decisions. For example, the practice of placing the burden of financing CHWs on the community has been shown to be broadly unsustainable and inequitable, but within the health-care system as a whole there may be possibilities for cross-subsidizing CHW programmes. Such opportunities can only be identified if a sector-wide approach is adopted. In order to make the appropriate decisions about financing options it is important to have better information about the costs of CHW programmes, and costing should be seen to be an important part of the planning, evaluation and replanning process.

The broader issue of sustaining CHW programmes must also be seen within the context of the whole health sector. In addressing the problems of sustainability, governments must not just consider how to finance the costs of programmes. They must also take steps to address the problems of task allocation and supervision already discussed. Even if funds are found, from whatever source, to support the wages of CHWs, CHW programmes will not be sustainable unless they provide – and are seen to provide – an effective service. This will only be possible if the links between CHWs and the other levels of the health system are reconsidered. Donors, too, need to consider their role in underpinning weak national programmes: withdrawal from provision of national training resources, for example, may force ministries of health to rethink policies regarding CHWs, such as the feasibility of training them locally. Diverting resources to help develop innovative local schemes, or to support new approaches to introducing incentives for supervision, may be more productive.

Our conclusions are clear. The concept of the CHW remains valuable, and much useful work can be done by CHWs. However, governments and donors must not be unrealistic in their expectations. In national programmes, as opposed to non-governmental CHW schemes, CHWs will almost always be limited to being extenders of services (not inconsiderable in itself) rather than agents of change for their communities. This does not mean that they will be unsympathetic to the needs of their communities, or that by being 'extra pairs of hands' they are not fulfilling a useful purpose. The concept stands. Having said that, we do not feel sanguine about the future of CHWs in national programmes unless real effort is put into enhancing their effectiveness so that they do not simply extend the possibility of contact with the health system, but also effectively tackle some of the community's health problems.

It is time for national governments and the international community to move away from insisting on a global or even national definition of the person and role of a CHW. National governments must foster local initiatives to address particular problems. They must provide a supportive context for such initiatives – for example, through developing field-based supervisory training schemes or by allowing non-monetary rewards to those working at the periphery (for example, time off in lieu of field trips, help with housing, and so on) and by channelling additional funds to the local level to strengthen the periphery. It is essential that the international community works with national governments in developing this context, recognizing existing resource constraints and not building up structures which cannot be sustained nationally. The key requirement is to put real effort into building both CHWs' skills and the support provided to them, and we have given some very specific ideas of where that effort could be focused.

However, our conclusions carry a more wide-reaching warning, not only for CHW programmes, but for the PHC approach itself. Unless the fragile primary health infrastructures, built up with so much enthusiasm in the 1960s and 1970s, are nurtured and protected, they will crumble in the face of economic strategies that are inimical to equity and state provision. It is, then, not only community health worker programmes that will face dissolution, but the whole primary health care approach. Our hope is that this will not be allowed to happen.

References

Abel-Smith, B. (1986). The world economic crisis. Part 1: repercussions on health. *Health Policy and Planning*, 1, 3, 202–13

Anderson, S. and Staugård, F. (1988). Traditional midwives in Botswana: strengthening links between women. *Health Policy and Planning*, 3, 1, 40–7.

Cherian, R. *et al.* (1988). Evaluation of simple clinical signs for the diagnosis of acute lower respiratory tract infections. *The Lancet* (II), 125–8.

Ennever, O. *et al.* (1988). The use of community health aides as perceived by their supervisors in Jamaica, East Indies (1987/88). *West Indies Medical Journal*, 37, 131–8.

Rifkin, S. and Walt, G. (1986). Why health improves: defining the issues concerning 'comprehensive primary health care' and 'selective primary health care'. *Social Science and Medicine*, 23, 559–66.

Ronsmans, C., Bennish, M.L. and Wierzba, R. (1988). Diagnosis and management of dysentery by community health workers. *The Lancet* (II), 552–5.

Unicef (1986; 1987). *The State of the World's Children*. Oxford University Press, Oxford.

Unicef (1988). *Adjustment with a Human Face*. Clarendon Press, Oxford.

Walt, G. (1988). CHWs: are national programmes in crisis? *Health Policy and Planning*, 3, 1, 1–21.

Index